The experts have spoken about *HeartSnark*!

"I pioneered historic, life-saving surgery for this??"

—Dr. Christiaan Barnard

"Sure, I invented the left ventricular assist device,
but I wish someone had invented
a 'lame author assist device.'"

—Dr. Michael DeBakey

"I'd trade my artificial heart for an artificial brain
if I could install it in this author."

—Dr. Robert Jarvik

"Why is there blood on my shoes?
Is it Kroenung's?"

—Dr. Jekyll

Also by Terry Kroenung
www.terrykroenungink.com

<u>Novels</u>
Brimstone and Lily: A Blade of Dubious Glory
Brimstone and Lily: Beware the Sword of Mirth
Jasper's Foul Tongue
Jasper's Magick Corset
Paragon of the Eccentric
Rapiers & Rogues
The Gaze of Zeus

<u>Drama</u>
The Three Musketeers
Coolness and Courage
Blood and Beauty
Gentle Rain

<u>Anthologies</u> (contributor)
Customs, Castles, and Kings, v. 2
Broken Links, Mended Lives
False Faces
Found

<u>Awards</u>
Colorado Gold Literary Award
Paragon of the Eccentric (winner)
Brimstone and Lily (finalist)

Independent Publishers Book Award
Brimstone and Lily (Bronze Medal)

Next Generation Indie Book Award
HeartSnark (finalist)

Colorado Short Story Contest
"The Day the Earth Couldn't Stand Still" (winner)

HeartSnark

A humorous account of my heart transplant,

featuring

Shakespearean strippers, bison meatloaf,
and urinal harems

Terry Kroenung

Additional Commentary

Janet Smith

RARE MOON PRESS
Longmont, Colorado

HeartSnark

Please visit terrykroenungink.com

DEDICATIONS

To my unknown donor and his family,
the English language doesn't have enough words to convey my love;
(don't worry, I'll take good care of him)

To my wife Janet,
If you hadn't been there,
I wouldn't have wanted to wake up anyway

And to my 5,000 Facebook friends,
most of whom have never even laid actual eyes on me;
without you this would have been exercise in misery, futility,
and unrelieved tedium.

(if the book is unrelieved tedium, well, that's on me)

"A light heart lives long."
Shakespeare, *Love's Labour's Lost*

"Let my liver rather heat with wine, than my heart cool with mortifying groans."
Shakespeare, *The Merchant of Venice*

"If I ever need a heart transplant, I want my ex-wife's. It's never been used."
Rodney Dangerfield

CONTENTS

ACKNOWLEDGEMENTS

Naturally, I need to thank a ton of people. If I left you out, my apologies.

Dr. Lynn Carlyle for recognizing that I was, in fact, one sick puppy, despite my naïve protestations to the contrary.

The Anschutz transplant doctors who made sure that I left the hospital on my own two feet: Amrut Ambardekar (head of the program, who overruled everyone else and said I should get a new heart, rather than go home); Eugene Wolfel (the avuncular one who ran point for the whole thing and kept me from freaking out); David Fullerton (the one who actually performed the surgery and who may be the calmest human being I ever met); and Michelle Knees (the resident who was there every day, demonstrating why she'll eventually be Surgeon-General).

Nancy Ireland, RN, and Nurse/Practitioner Emily Benton, who patiently explained everything a thousand times until our overwhelmed brains finally absorbed it all.

Kate Wilson, RN, my Transplant Coordinator, who must be wondering what she's done to deserve me, and my whole Transplant Team. You folks make this a (relative) breeze.

The Cardiac ICU Nursing Team for your unbelievable tenacity in putting up with my frequently literal crap for 17 days, and the Cardiac/Thoracic Surgical Unit for putting this thing in and ensuring that it works. It still seems like science-fiction.

My long-suffering wife Janet Smith, whom I love with every fiber of my being, (even the new fibers), and for whom I would donate every one of my organs.

My stepdaughter Alaena Prince, who needs some sort of 'I Ought to Get a Taxi License Out of This' medal for ferrying Janet hither and yon while all of this was happening.

Josh Bacca, for doing yeoman's work running every errand possible.

Maria Kuroshchepova, for possibly contributing more snarky comments to the original posts than anyone else, while also sending me multiple unanticipated goodie boxes.

Hey! Don't skip this!
(I worked all weekend on it)

Good for you, plucky reader! You took the high road and chose not to blast on by this part, which is actually pretty darned important, believe it or not. This Introduction clues you in on who I am, why this book exists, why it has a weird title, and why you should care. It will make the rest of the long slog more understandable and, therefore, endurable.

That's my story and I'm sticking to it.

On April 7, 2019, at the Anschutz Medical Center in Aurora, Colorado, they cut my heart out and tossed it in a trash can. Said receptacle, having some standards, promptly spit it back.

That's not strictly true. It was actually sliced and diced and sent to labs from the Mayo Clinic on down, because my ticker was *bizarre*. Not only didn't it work anymore, the high and mighty physicians involved turned out to be dead wrong about why. Keep this in mind, though: you never want your medical condition to be so rare that doctors from far and wide come to visit you in morbid fascination, visions of lucrative research grants cavorting in their heads.

This is the more-or-less humorous story of that heart transplant, from its origins two years before when I was fitted with a pacemaker, despite the doctor wondering why such a relatively young and healthy dude should need one, to six months into a hopefully glitch-free recovery from the transplant. Yes, you read that right. Humorous. Well, as humorous as my limited comedic skills could make it at the time. Thus the odd title for a subject that usually comes with the terms inspirational, courageous, uplifting, or tragic.

The core of the book is the running Facebook diary I kept every day as this insanity progressed. Both out of a natural proclivity toward black humor and out of a necessity to not go crazy and take a swan dive out of my hospital window (which would've made me an organ donor instead of a recipient), I took great pains to not act the victim or seek any sympathy at all. Instead, I tried to make as many snarky observations about my predicament as I could. To my amazement, my nearly 5,000 Facebook friends began responding to it as if it were some hit TV show. One even claimed that she was more into it than *Game of Thrones* (let's face it, my medical drama *was* less predictable than that ending). Not long after beginning the whole thing, people started suggesting that it should be a book. Many people. Repeatedly. Being an author of fantasy novels that no one reads, such clamor was a new experience for me. I wasn't too sure about it at the time, having more engrossing things on my mind like, you know, dying and all, but I kept an open mind. Later I had an open torso, too. After getting home in one piece (though the pieces were a bit different that before), I re-read the string of posts and agreed that something could be made of it all, but only if the facetious angle was the focus. There are already plenty of heart transplant books that aim to inspire or educate, written by people better qualified by temperament for that than I am.

But this is absolutely not intended to make light of the serious nature of the unfortunate donor's plight, and that of his family. Everything else is fair game for black humor here, but never that. I get to go on my merry way, miraculously saved, but they have an empty chair at the dinner table.

So this is the deal: what you have before you is the mostly unedited spewings I created from March 30, 2019, when I had to rush to the Emergency Room with runaway ventricular tachycardia (sounds like a Marvel villain) through the week of diagnosis, the surgery, the week of ICU recovery, and the five months of home recovery while composing this book. I chose not to go back and correct or prettify anything, unless there was a grievous factual error. It's an honest account of what I was experiencing and thinking in real time, no matter how lame. There are several pages of posts covering the time leading to the blessed event, to give a sense of the continuity to the thing. Those begin with April 22, 2017. Yes, Earth Day, that glorious homage to recycling. Appropriate, I think, considering. I had to back up so far because there was a significant foreshadowing event that summer. Yes, even more important than the year being designated as 'International Year of Sustainable Tourism for Development' by the UN.

Also included are the comments my Facebook friends made to these posts, along with my own, plus later comments on the comments, from my new perspective. It turns out that some of these people own a modicum of wit. Who knew? I wish this book could provide the hilarious videos and GIF's that often accompanied their comments. And by no means are all of their comments included here. That would have resulted in a book longer than Moby *Dick*, and with almost as many sharp implements and gore. Most of the responses were loving and supportive, so many, in fact, that it got a bit embarrassing on my end. Sincerity is not something I handle well. It overwhelmed me, frankly. I kept a few of those in, to communicate the flavor of it all, but I chiefly used the snarkier ones, since they matched the book's theme. Just keep in mind that the loving ones outnumbered the funny ones by at least 5 to 1.

Lastly, I have gone back through the posts/comments and added explanatory notes/reflections/so-called jokes.

Some biographical and medical items needed clarification, and at times I needed to give my honest thoughts about particular episodes. Hey, it can't all be comedy gold. My long-suffering wife, Janet (trust me, her suffering began long before my heart troubles) has done the same. With clever formatting, the various sections should be simple to keep straight.

I've chosen not to give you my biography in great detail, since it's not really necessary to understand the book and it's about as fascinating as a Congressional subcommittee report on turnip pricing. There will be brief explanations of episodes that you need to know so you won't be totally lost as to why I wrote a particular note or passage.

There's a semi-serious glossary of medical terms at the end. I **may** have snarked it up a bit.

So off you go, little fledglings, into the brave new world of my heart transplant. It's a deadly serious topic, yes, but just this once we can relax and laugh at modern medicine for the grand and glorious absurdity it can be…though you won't be laughing at the bills. Trust me on this.

WTF? This is just a bunch of Facebook posts

Just? Just a bunch of Facebook posts? You wound me, reader. These are the essential, the crucial, the vital Facebook posts. The *sine qua non* of posts, if you will (yeah, that Latin classes this book up enough that they'll add fifty cents to the cover price).

As mentioned in the Introduction that you *promised* me you wouldn't skip, the posts make up a sort of diary of my heart transplant experience, from the earliest cardiac rumblings two years before to post-op recovery at home. Plain text posts are my original observations and also the deathless comments on each by me and/or my friends. Anything in *italics* is what I added later, as explanations, clarifications, to help the reader understand enough to not hurl the book into the fireplace in frustration. If you still experience frustration after 4 hours, see your doctor. I also added even more of my deathless witticisms (see what I did there?).

Each major part of the book will begin with a general summary of people, things, events, etc. that are essential for comprehension. Biographical details, place names, events not overtly mentioned in the posts, medical terms, that sort of stuff. Inside of a particular post will be specific italicized notes on anything specific to that post, or my comments on the comments after the fact (you know you always think of that clever comeback after the conversation ends; this way I actually get to use those).

Now gird your loins, throw your manly shield before you, put in your mouthguard, and charge into Part 1.

To access the photos/videos/links:
www.terrykroenungink.com/246-2/

1) WELL, THAT SHOULD HAVE BEEN
MY *FIRST* HINT

April 22, 2017 to January 18, 2019

At the time Part 1 begins, my wife Janet and I are living in Loveland, Colorado, roughly an hour straight north of Denver. Small city, getting bigger as everybody and his idiot brother move here like it's the 1849 Gold Rush. Now housing prices are astronomical. Thanks, folks. Loveland's chiefly known for 2 unusual things: 1) it's the bronze sculpture capital of America (that's really a thing), full of artists, foundries, and sculpture gardens (mostly full of hyper-realistic cowboys, Native Americans, horses, buffalo, and children—abstraction need not apply) and 2) capitalizing on its name by remailing Valentine's Day cards from all over the country with the Loveland postmark. Tres romantique, non? Please don't tell those good people availing themselves of the service that the town was named after a 19th century railroad executive of that name. Sort of kills the magic.

Later in the section, we move to Longmont, less than 30 minutes south. It made for a shorter commute to my job teaching high school English. Janet is retired and living a life of scandalous decadence on her Social Security checks. This was made possible by those aforementioned insane housing prices, which got us lottery-level cash for our embarrassing hovel of a house. I said at the time that the other shoe would drop and my luck would turn. I like being on the right side of a housing bubble for once, but I also hate being right sometimes.

I teach English at Niwot High School. Don't pretend that you know where that is. I had to look it up to get to my job interview. The tiny town of the same name is mostly very economically/educationally fortunate folks working for IBM, Ball Aerospace, those sort of techie concerns. Chief Niwot of the southern Arapahoe supposedly said, "People seeing the beauty of this valley will want to stay, and their staying will be the undoing of the beauty." Since the town is the headquarters of Crocs Footwear, he may have been onto something.

For 15 years I've been known as the eccentric teacher there. Fair enough. I have very mild autism (Asperger Syndrome), teach Shakespeare by dressing up as him and instructing students in stage combat with real steel swords, get the class's attention with a fart gun from the Minions movie, sling wretched puns, and put stories I wrote on their essay tests for analysis. Throughout this book you'll see references to all of that, especially the Shakespeare and swordfighting stuff. I have degrees in theatre and fine arts, am a trained and experienced actor/playwright, and have won awards for my creative writing, mostly in the fantasy genre. That gets mentioned at times, too, along with my distance running and long-distance road cycling. The latter usually comes in the context of my falling off of the bike and getting an ambulance ride. In my defense, that only happened once and it was because the 30-year-old bike broke and tried to kill me (I did get a fancy-schmancy carbon fiber wonder-bike out of that, but when she saw the cost, my wife wanted to kill me). But at least they ran the siren. When they rushed me to the medical center pre-transplant, they outright refused when I asked. Nobody told the EMT's that you should honor a dying man's last request.

There are plenty of references, direct and oblique, to geeky stuff like superhero movies, Doctor Who, and Monty Python. Curling (I'm in a league) and cricket (I used to be in a league) will make appearance, too. And Eeyore. And a lot of politically liberal comments from me and my friends. If that last part bugs you, you might want to pass on this book.

2017

4/22/17
For Teacher Appreciation Week, I'd love for my former students to reply to this post and tell me how you are doing and what you are doing (school, job, career, family, etc.), include a pic if you like! Share one memory you have from my classroom. Even if you know that I know all about you — I still want to hear from you.

Jim: Well...I wasn't in your high-school class, but you did teach me stage combat and stage sword play. I recall a lesson from that, that can apply to humor in general: You can try a joke or a funny stunt three times, and it'll still be funny. The fourth time, it'll be dull. I also learned that when practicing the "kick me in the crotch" maneuver, to pick a fight partner who is NOT over a foot taller than you. (Talking about YOU, Kurt)
Kurt: Needed to apply following code:

New_Target_Height = (Original_Target_Height - 14 inches)

Call Kick (New_Target_Height)

Next time I'll run the subroutine!

Jim: Yes, please. And do some unit-testing on yourself, first.

Dai: But by the tenth time it's hilarious again.

Taryn: Let's see. I think it was my junior year of high school and you assigned extra credit to the students if they bought a copy of *Brimstone and Lily* and had you sign it at Borders. Another memory was when you assigned a Write Like Edgar Allan Poe paper. And mine ended up in the school Literary Journal. I am currently living in Loveland with my future husband, working two jobs and going to school to major in Psychology.

'Brimstone and Lily' was my first novel, a sort of swords-and-sorcery 'Huck Finn.' The assignment was to get students into a bookstore, not to intimidate them into buying the book at my author event. For those too young to remember, a bookstore was a place where people would take their physical selves and actually obtain reading matter that didn't have batteries. Border's was a major chain of such places, back in the Before

Times.

Ellie: Hey! I'm finishing my first year of college at CU Boulder! Going into business. I miss helping with Shakespeare!

For some reason Coloradans call the University of Colorado CU. In Illinois, where I was born, we called the University of Illinois the U of I. That CU isn't called the U of C, or even UC, just goes to show how much weed is circulating here. Adding to the weirdness, my transplant was at the university teaching hospital, which they call UC Medical Center.

Laura: You taught me how to act and sword fight so here goes: married and a high school teacher.

Joshua: I've only been out of high school a year and I've already been tazed four times, been to jail, and bit a cop...so things are going great.

Josh: I'm currently in N.C. cooking at a country club, and I brought my rapier with me just in case.

Josh is my chief stage combat assistant and a professional chef. I'm guessing when you order shish kabob at his restaurant, it gets your attention.

4/23/17
25 miles on the bike for Willie Shakes' birthday, climbing up to Carter Lake (12% hill, 3 miles, woo-hoo!).

Me: No, I didn't wear the doublet and ruff. Sorry to disappoint.

FYI, I have at least half a dozen Elizabethan doublets. Don't you?

5/25/17
And that's Year 26 of teaching in the can. Signed, sealed, and delivered. I'm outta here (for 11 weeks, anyway).

And off to a disturbingly eventful summer.

6/11/17
6 dizzy spells walking the dog, nearly all requiring putting a hand on the ground so that I didn't fall clear over. Some medical genius better fix this crap. NEVER happens running or biking. Elevated pulse seems to prevent it. #losingmysenseofhumor

Just to show you how clueless somebody with a Mensa membership can be, I'd been ignoring the dizzy spells for months. When I couldn't do that anymore, I tried self-treatment: changes to diet, checking the house, car, and school for allergens or toxins, adjusting my hypothyroid meds…anything but going to see an actual trained professional. Looking back, there had been a couple of brief episodes at school in the preceding year or more, which I had put down to transient minor colds, etc. A couple of times a school secretary said I looked bad and should she drive me home? I didn't take her up on it. After the transplant, she made sure I remembered it. Got a little smug about her diagnostic skills, she did. Okay, okay, Michelle. You were right. Happy now?

So I saw my family practice doctor, who stuck a Holter monitor on me for a week. This is an irritating portable device that hangs around your neck, with several adhesive leads sucking up your cardiac vital signs and hurling them across the ether so your doctor can see what's up. What he failed to mention was that the info also went to a remote company whose job it was to alert me via phone that I was having a cardiac episode, nearly always waking me out of a sound sleep. In every one of those instances I felt perfectly fine and asymptomatic, leading me to curse their very existence. Okay, okay, Michelle. You were right. Happy now?

6/20/17
I've kept a log for the past 11 days and I'm averaging 6 dizzy/near-fainting spells a day. 7 this morning during one dog walk. That's not counting all of the times when the heart monitor people called at 3 a.m. to tell me that my heart stopped for 6-10 seconds. #reallydon'twantafreakingpacemaker

(Janet) The first time the phone rang at 3am, we both nearly hit the ceiling. Could have had double heart attacks!

Laura: I'm on my third pacemaker. They aren't that bad and they do help a lot. If you want to ask me about it, let me know. I've had one since I was 8, now I'm 42. I'd be dead without it.

Me: They haven't mentioned the word 'dead' quite yet, but I could always keel over and fracture my skull on something, like William Holden did.

Me: So long as I can still sword fight, run races, and climb insane hills on the bike, I could resign myself to it.

Laura: Well, my heart was going down below 20/30 beats a minute while sleeping at age 7/8 and if it kept slowing down it would finally just stop.

Me: Mine's not quite that low yet. Cardio guy says all of the workouts may actually make it worse, because that naturally slows it all down with the improved fitness. Echocardiogram says the ticker is otherwise a splendid specimen.

Me: How long do the batteries last?

Insert your off-color joke here: _____.

Laura: Good luck. My first lasted forever, but it was implanted in 1982. The second just over 9 years. The third I had put in on Jan 15, 2009 and they say at least 2 more years.

Me: How much of a pain is going to be to put in? Asking for a friend.

Laura: Not that bad. Some pain pills, a week or so of rest and that was it. No driving or lifting things above my head for a couple of weeks. Honestly, my hernia surgery was much worse.

M Cid: Oh, my dear friend. Do everything to keep yourself well.

Me: I plan on lingering for enough decades that your life will be a hellscape, Mikey.

6/20/17
Good news: this #$@! heart monitor comes off today. Woo-hoo!

Bad news: they just called and said I was having 'concerning' readings all flipping night.

Janet: At least they were kind enough not to call at 3:00 am.

Dave: Ugh, I'm sorry. I hated the Holter monitor.

Me: It's off. Free at last!

Jim: No more power pasties?

6/22/17
It's more than a little disturbing to see your Fitbit suddenly stop registering your pulse...repeatedly. Thus the concern of multiple doctors lately. Or maybe I really am a heartless bastard.

Serge: Remember...the Tin Man thought he had no heart either, but did have one all along.

If my chest starts to echo, I'll take up heavy drinking. I already need an oil can for my arthritic joints. (interestingly, a heart sonogram is called an echo)

Me: Looks like it was trying to tell me something (typed from a hospital bed the next day).

6/23/17
Had 13 dizzy spells today and my doctor freaked when he saw the week's heart monitor summary. So did the cardiologist. He wouldn't let me leave the hospital. Says I've been flatlining. This ticker could just stop. So guess who's getting a shiny new pacemaker tomorrow morning? #andhow'syourweekend?

(Janet) I took the call from the doctor's office and he was telling the nurse to tell me that he was "very concerned" and that we needed to get to the cardiologist's office pronto. Dr. Elmo has a temperament that does not generally exhibit concern, so off to the hospital we went.

That's right, my doctor was named Elmo. And he did tickle me...in unmentionable places.

Hope: What is the recovery time?

Me: Here till Sunday morning. We're still going to your wedding. I won't be dancing, though.

Garalt: Most people dramatise this as *King Lear*, but here you are playing it like *As You Like It*. Well played, sir.

Well, that is the point of this book, after all: Laughing in the Face of Death. Or snickering, at least.

Me: If I go all *Titus Andronicus*, that'll be the time to worry.

If you aren't familiar with Shakespeare's 'Titus Andronicus,' check it out. Just don't blame me if you keel over from all of the judicial amputations, rapes, murders, and baking people into pies to serve to their mother.

Garalt: Just as long as it isn't *Measure for Measure*. I'd have to evacuate Janet.

Another Shakespeare gem, where a temporary city administrator tries to extort sex from a virgin nun by threatening to behead her brother for the crime of — get this — fornication.

Hope: Hey, if Bexa is potentially still coming 9+ months pregnant, I don't expect a heart surgery to stop you. (TOTALLY KIDDING)

Mark: Thinking about you, my friend. "It's just a flesh wound..."

Ding-ding-ding! And there's our first Monty Python allusion.

Me: And 2 electrodes implanted in my beating heart.

Heather: Good luck tomorrow. Pick out a pretty one.

Not sure how pretty it was, but the guy from Boston Scientific who assisted in the Catheter Lab claimed it was the 'Ferrari of pacemakers.' You can safely go through an MRI machine with it.

Well, this isn't how I thought my weekend would go. (photo 1)

My first night in a hospital since the removal of my appendix in 2013. Then it was gangrene and peritonitis. I never go halfway with my medical issues.

Julie: Maybe the therapy dogs will come by.

Valerie: Perhaps they can install a pacemaker in your brain to send electrical impulses directly into your grey matter. Like a steady electroshock therapy. Then, hand me the controller.

M Cid: You make baby Jesus cry.

Valerie: We all make Baby Jesus cry.
Me: But then, so does colic.

At the time I was in a mood to slap the bejeesus out of Jesus.

M Cid: I was just thinking, Terry, all this trouble started when you tried exercising. Exercising will just get you into trouble. If I were you, I'd focus on eating greasy fried food and watching Judge Judy all day.

Me: It all started after I friended you on FB. Coincidence? I think not.

Sarah: First step to bionic man! Happy recovery.

It's no fun being bionic if you can't jump over tall obstacles with that do-do-do-do music playing.

Garalt: Yeah, it always has to happen in leisure time. Sheesh! You just got off for the summer. Talk about not taking advantage of workplace legislation. On the bright side...Obamacare is still in effect, right?

Luckily, I discovered that my school district insurance was first-rate. Good thing. Wouldn't have wanted to go into hiding when the pacemaker repo men showed up.

(Janet) It may be first-rate now, but at the time they were changing companies and HRA's, so I spent almost a full year on the phone trying to get things straightened out. The hospital billing department didn't help. The UC Health system we are in now and the school insurance is much better coordinated.

Con: My pulse alarm just went off when it hit 37 BPM.
Pro: The night nurse is photogenic.

Yeah, I have a Y chromosome. Sue me.

Harriet: Well, that might get your pulse going, but she can't stay there all night!

John: Before my pacemaker, I could get my pulse down to 34 in the evening.

Me: I have the same problem. I can run 5 miles, bike until my pulse hits 170 (did that yesterday), but might expire in my sleep.

Me: Mine went down to 34 tonight and everybody freaked.

Hope: Pro tip, if it is like the monitor I had, and you have to unplug it to go to the bathroom, remember to plug it back in or the battery dies and it registers no heartbeat.

Me: There's no 'going' anywhere. I have to stand next to the bed and fill a bottle. Not allowed to move anywhere else.

Yeah, that piddling into a bottle thing is practically a running theme in this book. Could've been worse. Could've been daily stool samples.

Apparently, U.S. Doctors put in 100,000 pacemakers a year. My doctor implants 5 a week. Does NOBODY's freaking heart work in this country? #seemslikeadesignflaw.

Not sure if they recycled mine to a Third World nation after the transplant or if the military has it for a bomb fuse.

Hoping they give me video of my pacemaker surgery and echocardiogram, so I can appall my students in August. I showed them my brain scan years ago. That was fun.

My doctor at the time said I had a 'pristine' brain. I took that to mean it was free of concerning stuff. My so-called friends took it to mean it was free of coherent thought.

An echocardiogram is an ultrasound of your heart. It can detect all sorts of issues. I have no idea how the techs read them. To me they just look like John Hurt's chest before the alien bursts out.

Laura: I can always send you a pic of my first pacemaker. It was in me for 18 years.

Taryn: I don't think you ever showed the class of 2010 your brain scans.

Now I don't where that disc went. Probably ended up in a pristine trash can.

Ellie: I'd love to see the video of the surgery and echo if you have it!

6/24/17
Man, when your heart rate drops down to 28 and gets big gaps in it at 3 a.m., alarms go off and nurses come running.

Janet: What is it about 3 a.m. that makes your heart stop?

Probably running systems diagnostics...or smoking weed out on the quad of the hippocampus.

Veronica: I mean, there are easier ways to get the nurses to visit.

Jeez, I'm literally hooked up to the machine that goes "ping!"

And there's our second Python reference, from the birthing scene in 'The Meaning of Life.'

Julia: Just hope it keeps going "ping."

Bren: "Ah, I see you have the machine that goes ping. This is my favorite. You see we lease it back from the company we sold it to and that way it comes under the monthly current budget and not the capital account."

Quoting from the movie. The check's in the mail, Messers. Cleese, Palin, et al.

So, if you want a real thrill, watch your hospital heart monitor flash

red, sound an alarm, and read 0. That happened more than once last night. #morefunthanthelawallows

I literally watched myself flatline for 10 seconds on the monitor. That gets your attention in a hurry. Then the heart's backup electrical system would kick in before I could pass out and everybody could relax...until it happened again...and again.

Decades of hard-core running/biking, vegetarian diet, fish oil capsules, etc., and I STILL end up with freaking heart failure. #sortofpissedoff

One imagines brawny ladies in kerchiefs and aprons, wring out fish like washcloths to get the oil. One also hopes that's not how they make baby oil.

Linda: My mum, 93 this week, smoked plenty a day until 87, never exercised and ate everything she wanted including cholesterol-inducing full-fat cream and milk, has just got heart failure. Yes, I know it's not fair!

Yulonda: Well, I'm gonna eat this double stack bacon sandwich with this news. Thanks, Terry!! Good luck today.

Gloria: Yep! Your destiny lies in the stars, not fish oil.

You know, if I have to be bionic, I'd rather have the telescope eye, tank tread feet, and rotating autocannon arm. #justapacemaker

Scott: It all starts somewhere. I mean, Darth Vader's armor basically was a pimped-out iron lung.

They're hauling me off in 15 or 20 minutes for the Grand Implantation. The hotshot doctor says he's tuning the pacemaker for Sports mode.

Spoiler: He did not.

Dean: It has a nice beat. I can dance to it. I give it a 100.

M Cid: Can I have the afterbirth? It's for science!
Don't you go creating a Master Race again, Mikey. That didn't work out so well last time.

Carol: When my husband got his, I asked for a remote for the defibrillator function. Who needs a Taser?

I nearly got one of those. I was 10 minutes from surgery this year when they cancelled it and stuck a new heart in me instead. Couldn't there have been some sort of middle ground, like a pneumatic hand-squeezed vest that I could use to pump myself up?

Fun fact: TASER stands for Tom Swift's Electric Rifle. Seriously. Now there's an obscure allusion on their part.

Adam: Ask him to tune it to Radio 4.

Ah, British radio. I have friends on nearly every continent. Of my nearly 5,000 friends on Facebook, I personally know/have been in the company of less than 10%. It's a writer thing, accumulating fellow authors. I hope to collect the whole set and win a stuffed panda toy or something.

Dave: You will be Locutus of Borg! F**k Patrick Stewart!!!

And now we've moved on to 'Star Trek' (when Patrick Stewart was made into a Borg; better than 'Star Search', anyway.

(Janet) Terry is done with surgery and is fine!

(update) Well, fine-ISH.

Heather: Are you going to bike yourself home?

M Cid: Terry who?

Janet: He's having some chest pain, so they are going to do a chest X-ray.

Kelly: Is that normal?

Janet: Not really, which is why they are checking.

Yeah, you know what's coming. A 'plot complication' that's a literal complication.

(Janet) The doctor was thinking that Terry would be out of here by 5pm. With the chest pain, they are doing tests.

Mark: They just had his chest open and they're wondering why he is having chest pain??

FYI, you don't really 'open' the chest to implant a pacemaker. You make a 3-inch incision in the left chest just south of the collarbone, then run 2 electrical wires into the right ventricle and right atrium by punching a hole in a big vein under your collarbone. Those are harpooned or screwed into the inside of the heart wall. The other end of the wires attach to a tiny wonder-computer the size of a pocket watch, which is tucked into the hole you just made under the skin. They call it 'minimally invasive', which is what you say when it isn't happening to you.

I imagine my doctor spearing my right ventricle and screaming, "From Hell's heart I stab at thee!" That makes him a…Herman Melvillain.

Janet: Doctor isn't sure what is going on.

Jim: Doctor left his game controller inside?

*Oh, **that's** why I keep getting chased by giant Pac-men. God thing he wasn't into 'Grand Theft Auto.'*

Me: I suggested he left a wrench in there. He said they're crazy careful about that sort of thing now. Though he did confess to leaving a sponge in some poor lady in med school.

And she wasn't even a patient.

Me: Redoing the whole operation in 2 hours. He thinks one of the electrodes punctured the heart wall a bit too far.

And it came out the other side. Less than a 1% chance. Doctor said it was only the third time in his career that it'd happened. If you saw how vague the fluoroscope image is that they go by, you'd wonder that anybody survives.

Well, the 'simple textbook pacemaker operation' went sideways in a hurry. The operation itself went swimmingly, the surgeon said. But back in the room, my chest behind the sternum started to hurt like the wrath of god with every breath. Not part of the plan. So they sent me down for an x-ray. It got worse on the way back. In my room when they tried to put me back in the bed, my BP plummeted to 67/40 and I passed out. Everybody freaked and I was swarmed by med people. Another echocardiogram showed no punctures, swelling, or fluid, so the surgeon was puzzled. Pacemaker's working perfectly. Naturally, my 5 p.m. checkout isn't happening now. Here overnight while they see if it all calms down on its own. Hurts less now. Might just be inflammation from the electrodes. My heart might be pissed at the indignity.

UPDATE: in 2 hours I'm getting the whole operation again.

Me: BP back up to 100/60 (low normal).

Mark: Terry, maybe your next book should be your autobiography——this is good stuff! Get better and get out of there, pal!

Me: 123/63 now. That's good. Chest pain's back some. Who knew that getting stabbed in the heart would hurt? #Draculaknew

Who knew that the day would come when I'd laugh uproariously at that wimpy chest pain?

KT: Pacemakers can be weird. My Mom's once showed she was dead for five hours one night.

And soon bloodless corpses started cropping up in her neighborhood. #getthegarlic

Garalt: Maybe avoid odd years in the future? Consider cryopods.

A reference to my penchant for having near-death experiences happen in odd-numbered years. 2011: bike wreck, head-first straight down onto pavement. Saved by helmet. Ambulance ride. 2013: the already-mentioned gangrenous appendix. 2015: heat stress on my bike climbing a mountain with a 13% grade. Another ambulance, and a great 4th of July experience. 2017: well, you know about that one. And you can probably guess *about 2019. This year I had a *SPOILER*.*

♫ **"Hello, Percocet, my old friend..."**

Yes, this joke will be recycled here in 2 years. No point in re-inventing the wheel.

Janet: Is that the good stuff?

Me: No, the really good stuff goes straight into the IV.

Garalt: ♫ "Just the soooound…of monitors…"

Me: You have no idea. If I never hear another electronic noise...

Garalt: Yeah, electro is so over for you. I'll tell Will-I-Am.

Perry: It's okay, Kraftwerk are pretty boring, really.

Alaena: Glad to see you are in the land of the living. Feeling any better this morning?

Me: Not a lot. Chest hurts with the very pulse and breath. Doctor thinks a wire went in too deep. I'm about to get the whole operation again to fix it.
Mark: Well, then, I'd ask for a discount on your bill! WTH?

6/25/17
Breaking pacemaker news: in 2 hours they have to redo the whole operation. Doctor thinks one of the electrodes went in too deep and actually penetrated through the heart wall a tiny bit (it's essentially a little electrified harpoon). So he has to pull them both out and jab them in someplace else. At least the pacemaker signal works beautifully. All of the arrhythmias and stoppages are gone. It just hurts like a freaking heart attack.

So: my odd-numbered-year luck (or lack of it) holds.

Veronica: Shit. *shakes fist at doctor for not doing it right*

Me: It's as much art as science. The image he had to work from is hardly clear. This guy is actually really good.

Veronica: I can still shake my fist.

Rebecca: There you go blaming X-ray, we always get the blame.

Rebecca was a radiologist (oh, excuse me, she insists on 'radiological technologist') for 40 years. You'll see as you read the whole book that she believes that this somehow makes her an expert on the subject. Some people…

Me: For everybody cursing the doctor: he's top-drawer (does 4 or 5 of these a WEEK) and was pro enough to immediately see the new problem. The image he has to use to precisely implant wires into a beating heart looks like a cat's hairball. I'm amazed pacemakers work at all.

Michelle: Are they giving you an OR punch card?

Me: I suggested that. They laughed.

But I did end up with a 2-for-1 special.

M Cid: I tell you what — all this money you're wasting on these quacks? LET ME do the surgery. I have more than enough knives, and I'll only charge you $50. So, what's the problem anyway? Is it a sex change you're going through? No problem.

Me: Stay away from me with those things or I'll change YOUR sex.

Heather: You broke it already?

Me: "To beat or not to beat, that is the question…"

Me: Off to the races. Hoping this is the last one.

That's what they need to liven miserable hospital stays: to-the-death gurney races. 'Now playing, 'Med Max Beyond Thunderdome'!"

Lottie: Oh, my GOD — poor you. You are so sweetly upbeat about all this. XX

Beth: Though I'm sorry for your pain, your play-by-play is certainly making this entertaining to hear about.

"Kroenung's up to bat, runners in scoring position, 2 outs, the Grim Reaper on the mound..."

Jilly: Be sure to have the device turned on when you get the bill!!

'American (Pacemaker) Horror Show' update (gruesome details):

Friday—serious dizzy spells, over a dozen in one morning. Family doctor 'very concerned', insists I see cardiologist. Cardio guy so concerned he forces me into a hospital bed, saying my heart has been stopping. All that night he's proven right, as I constantly, though briefly, flatline. I disbelieve this, having just climbed a 13% gradient on my bike.

Saturday—surgeon agrees with other doctors, schedules me for an immediate pacemaker. Not a serious procedure nowadays. He does 5 of them a week. Promises that I'll be home for dinner that day and back biking in 2 weeks. That seems to be true. Operation goes swimmingly (the OR techs joke about pizza lunch at Domino's). The arrhythmias utterly cease. But I have sharp pain behind my sternum (not normal). They send me down for a routine chest x-ray to see what's up. When I come back to my room, my blood pressure crashes from 110/70 to 67/40. I pass out and start to go into shock. Lots of medical professionals swarm me and bring me back. Echocardiogram shows nothing major. I have to stay in the ICU again while decisions are made.

Sunday—surgeon says the electrode he implanted has penetrated the heart wall enough to cause fluid leakage into the pericardium. He has to redo the whole pacemaker implantation. Only the third time he's ever had that happen. All will be well, he says. New operation goes perfectly, pain gone, rhythm fine.

BUT...as soon as I get back in my room, I crash again. Much worse. Complete unconsciousness, shaking, eyes rolled up in my head. BP drops to 50/30! They call an emergency code, in comes the crash cart and defibrillator (though that didn't get used). Room swarmed with doctors and nurses again. I wake to see a bunch of epically serious faces. It's like a movie from the POV of the dead guy who's about to start haunting people until he learns a Very Important Lesson. I'm completely lost as to what's going on. They stabilize me and do another echocardiogram. Some fluid building up around the heart from the first electrode problem, pushing on the heart. Apparently, this is 'VERY BAD.' In another nanosecond a gazillion emergency people in scrubs are literally running my bed into the Cath Lab (after telling Janet to give me a potential final kiss), where they performed pericardiocentesis (in plain language: a huge freaking needle is punched way into my chest and heart with NO anesthesia). Words cannot express how much this hurt.

When I made the predictable distressed noises as it went in, he said, trying to be reassuring, "I know." No, you don't, dude. It's never been done to you, has it?

And it was sustained, too. They pulled 12 ounces of fluid. Then they put in a drain to let any more get out while they put a watch on me. Nobody's telling jokes this time.

Now—vitals all fine again, original arrhythmias still fixed, no fluid building up. The original hole that caused the problem seems to have begun healing already. But they're keeping me here until probably Tuesday, to make sure. And the drain they installed hurts EXACTLY like the problem it's intended to fix. Thank god for whatever painkiller just went into my IV.

3 am — heart pain so bad I can only take the smallest of catch breaths. Every time I do it feels like swallowing razors. My whimpering draws nurses who give me stuff in the IV to dull it. But I wake up delirious, seeing no one, still in agony and literally crying for help. It was like my life was being stage-managed by Kafka, with special effects by Satan.

Then the surgeon came in and took out the tubes. He said that they were in just about every ventricle.

Words fail me.

Well, clearly not. That was a 650-word post.

FYI, dying feels like nausea and fainting at the same time, with an acidic aftertaste. I don't recommend it.

(Janet) After the second try at implanting the leads, they brought Terry back to the room. He wanted a drink of water and seemed fine until his eyes rolled up and he passed out. There wasn't a nurse or doctor in the immediate area and after pushing the call button, I went out into the hallway and shouted for someone. Finally, a crew was in the room trying to revive him. They wheeled him through the labyrinth to surgery with me following. One of the doctors told me to kiss him goodbye. What??? This was supposed to be a quickie 5-hour procedure and he's in danger of expiring? After they drained out the heart, the doctor came in and explained that if the hole didn't close up, they'd have to take him to Greeley and patch the hole with open heart surgery. Thankfully, that wasn't necessary...yet. Give it another 20 months.

Tana-Lee: That is one hell of a book hook! You have me on the edge of my seat here.

Hopefully not a toilet seat.

Valerie: Sounds like good reasons to have our consciousnesses transferred into robots.

Nope. Can't do it. Those 3 Laws of Robotics are too restrictive. I reserve the right to let harm come to a human...probably a doctor.

Alaena: The fact that you are writing mini-novels already is a good sign. Had me fretting today.

Susan: Holy crap! What a terrifying experience! And yet, your writing is so captivating — I am literally hanging on every word — that I am in awe.

Jami: I'm impressed that you can do these updates so lucidly!!

That makes two of us.

Caity: This sounds almost Shakespearean. So many plot twists.

Pro tip for all humans: you NEVER want your life to be Shakespearean.

Moshe: I hope all this misery at least entities you to skip Purgatory when your time is really up, decades from now.

Skip Purgatory? What the, um, Hell do you think **this** *is???*

Jennifer: No, words certainly did not fail you.

Christine: Wow, pericardial tamponade, if I remember my terminology correctly. Now you have a new word of the day for your students.

Correct! You win a coupon to the hospital cafeteria for a free Jello cup.

Pericardial tamponade means that the tough sac surrounding the heart fills up with fluid, usually blood, and smothers the heart action like an anaconda. If it happens slowly, the pericardium can safely hold 2 liters (!). But if it's rapid, like mine, a mere 200 ml can kill you. I had nearly twice that, because that's how I roll.

Kathleen: Words fail me at how you are able to write this posting and in such a deliverable way. Gawd!

Deborah: You're taking this whole Shakespearean drama thing a little too far! Fie! Fie! Draw thy sword and fight like you mean it!

'I am slain!'

Garalt: Three ops, two flatlines....your insurer is going to LOVE you.

Little did we know much my insurer was eventually going to hate me. It was a naïve, simpler time.

Kristi: OK! Enough already! Are you trying out ideas for a book?!

Well, duh!

Julie: You can dial it back a little, you've already attained your surgeon's "most interesting patient" status.

Again, we were clueless about just how Chinese Curse Level my 'interesting' would get.

Christina: Holy crap! You have me on the edge of my seat!

Mark: "Words fail me" ?? For an author, that can be serious!! ;)

Depends. If only that '50 Shades of Grey' chick had experienced such a failure.

"To beat or not to beat, that is the question..."
From Shakespeare's little-known cardiac opus, *'King Henry I. V.'*

Christine: Yup, snark's still there, you'll be fine. (((((hugs)))))

Liana: It's the drugs!

Sorry, the bad jokes are a pre-existing condition.

Jennifer: Serious as a heart attack.

Mark: So long as it's not coming from under the floorboards.

That's a Poe excuse for an allusion.

6/26/17
(Janet) Terry's blood pressure is better and they took out the drainage tube. He is wiped out by four operations in two days. Sleeping a little now. They will be watching carefully. Need to watch for fluid build-up and infection.

Only one drainage tube. Later I'd sigh wistfully for only the one, as my current 9 scars attest.

(Janet) Sleeping. (photo 2)

Looks like I'm laid out for the wake.

Hope: With a fancy hat no less.

Janet: I brought him his Eeyore hat when they wrapped his head in a towel.

Yeah, Eeyore is a thing. No idea why or how, it just happened. My classroom has over

25 versions, from singing ones to change purses to one that sucks on a strawberry and burps. Did I mention that I'm an actual adult person?

Simple outpatient procedure turn into hellish 4-night hospital nightmare. Or, as Shakespeare would call it: ***Rogue 1: A Midsummer Night's Shitshow.***

Me: Also apropos: "Other than that, Mrs. Lincoln, how'd you like the play?"

Hope: Progress?

Me: Well, they've stopped cutting on me and puncturing me with Joseph Mengle's hand-me-down needles. Still hurts to breathe. But the heart rhythm's now perfect. No stoppages.

Sharon: Shit show? Why not write a play?

No $ in it. I'll take my chances in the lucrative, risk-free world of book publishing instead.

It occurs to me that a theatre critic's job is, um, cast-rating.

Dave: I was hearing you in my head singing Janis Joplin. "Take another piece of my heart!"

M Cid: My kingdom for a lobotomy!

Oh, I'll lobotomize you for free, Mikey. What are friends for?

ICU, how do I love thee? Let me count the ways... (photo 3)

Fred: The deep anal probe is next, Mr. Kroenung.

Ah! I see the Billing Department is here. Is the Vaseline extra?

Me: That would be preferable to Sunday's deep heart probe without benefit of anesthesia.

Mario: I hope you're not there 21 days. That would be an awkward photo.

Hands, feet, nose, right? Why, did you have something else in mind for #21?

Going home soon! (photo 4)

I look like I'm going to a mental home, though.

6/27/17
Ladies and gentlemen, the tragic cardiac patient is now at home on his own couch.

Update: if the fever gets any worse, I'll have to go back.

That update is what we in the pro writing biz call 'foreshadowing.'

Cindi: The "lucky" cardiac patient.

Tina: NO dancing on tables, ya hear?

Not for free, anyhow. "Make it rain!"

Russell: So, an end to the heartache and the thousand natural shocks that flesh is heir to? Hope so. Get well soon!

*Alas, wrong on both counts, ache **and** shocks, as you'll see.*

Sharon: Bravo, bravo! Message to the audience...there will be no repeat performance! The tragedy has now become a comedy of errors! King Lear is resting on his couch rather than his throne (unless he has to go potty) and is not wearing that funky prairie dress but, alas, his robe...hail to the king! He lives!

All correct, save for the repeat performance bit. This ended being a long run, not a one-night special event.

I have actually played King Lear, in 2012. Grew out the gray beard for 4 months. Looked like my late dad. Janet ordered me to never do that again.

Marion: Glad you're out. Oh, and BTW, there's probably a mystery bill which you'll get in several months. You'll pay it full, and this will be followed up anyway a few months later with another mystery bill for $6.78, which will be pursued relentlessly.

The total for the first 6 months of 2019 was $1.9 million.

Maria: The re-implanting went well, then?

Me: Well, after they stabbed me with a ginormous heart needle and agonizingly drained 12 ounces of fluid that was drowning it and sending me into shock, yeah. Good times.

Ah, the joys of non-stop IV's in the ICU. They did both arms, FYI. (photo 5)

My 2019 self: You call that IV bruising? Here, hold my beer!

Scott: Ouch, damn spot!

Hope: Ouch! Make sure to start flexing it. I got rigor in my arm from too much IV.

Tina: Terry, during my odyssey with breast cancer, they used up both arms with bloodwork/transfusions and had to go between my fingers and toes. Ouch!

6/28/17
The fever seems to have broken.

Like my own birth, that proved to be premature.
Janet: It was a rough night with the fever almost hitting the call the doctor point but it broke finally and he's a little better now. For some reason they only gave him Ibuprofen and no antibiotics.

Hard as this long unanticipated hospital weekend was on me, it was worse on my poor honeybunch. All I had to do was lie there and

drool. She had to watch me get wheeled off to 3 operating rooms and get revived on the bed twice.

Janet: Standing next to your hubby, handing him a cup of water and immediately seeing his eyes roll up while he passes out and having to shout for nurses to come is not something I care to see again. And then following the bed down to the OR where one of the doctors says to give him a kiss before they wheel him in. What??? This was supposed to be an easy peasy slap-in-the-pacemaker thing, not life-threatening surgery!

Jim: You heal up, then you get to take care of your lady, very nice dinner, a drink, and a very heartfelt thank you!!

6/29/17
First shower in a week, what with all of the hospital hullabaloo and restrictions on the pacemaker incision. And I've walked 2 miles today without dizzy spells or cardiac events. #it'sthelittlethings.

10,000 steps and 5 miles today, according to the Fitbit. Woo-hoo!

Kate: Wow, you don't mess around with recovery!!!

Janet: I'm sure it was too much too soon.

Christine: Terry, if you cause yourself to relapse, I will come to your hospital room, pull the pacemaker from your still-beating heart with my bare hands, flog you with it, and reinsert it, all sans anesthesia. *scowls fiercely*

You make that sound like it's a bad thing.

7/1/17
Just sayin'. (photo 6)

Me: The pacemaker is under the word 'wife'. Whatever that means.

Today is my 'weekiversary' of being a cyborg. So we're off to enrich the local restaurateurs. If we're lucky, I'll score free dessert with my sorry hospital tale. #can'thurttotry

M CiD: Wait - you're still alive? sigh. I suppose I need to cancel that wreath order I was sending to Janet.

We'll use it on our front door as a Christmas wreath until you're inevitably shot by a jealous husband, then you'll get it back with a nice note.

Janet: Do cyborgs eat food?

Only the iron-rich stuff and um, electro-lytes.

Medical alert bracelet duly ordered. Didn't think I'd ever have to do THAT.

Garalt: Pretend it's an ironic Fitbit.

Pretend?

David: Do they have ones for "bad attitude?"

Me: Yeah. Not a bracelet, though. For me, that would be a tattoo.

7/5/17
Jogged about 50 meters today, just to see if I fell down dead post-pacemaker. FYI: I didn't. #don'ttellmycardiologist

Mandy: *starts dialing*

Careful, that'll be a pricey call from Wales.

Christine: Remember Janet does not have a pacemaker, so try not to stop her heart with your shenanigans.

Terry W.: Your doctor is going to have a heart attack.

Couldn't happen to a nicer guy.

7/7/17
Yet another thing I'd never thought I'd have to acquire: furry shoulder pads on my seat belt to cushion the pacemaker.

Me: At least they're "tell me about the rabbits, George" soft.

Fiona: When are you going to upgrade to arc reactor? *(the glowy thing in Iron Man's chest)*

Any day now. And nothing else. I'll be, um, Stark naked.

Jogged a half-mile with no ill effects from being a cyborg. And by 'jog', I mean putting one foot in front of the other like I'm 100 years old, underwater, towing a dump truck.

Felt like I was trying to run up a 30% hill wearing Marley's chains.

Tina: Don't feel bad: I have days like that, where the neighbors are betting whether I'll make it in the house!

What odds are you offering? I have medical bills to pay.

Andrew: We shall start having to call you Steve. Unless you prefer Mr. Austin?

Oblique reference to a 70's TV show. Try to keep up.

Garalt: I know US medical care is expensive, but $6 million?

Scott: That's why Steve Austin had to do all those missions; he'd blown past his lifetime cap.

7/8/17
Well, this sucks out loud.

Fever and infection, so it's back into the #%*! hospital again, for at least one night, so they can give me industrial-grade antibiotics. At least there's no current plan for scalpels and heart needles, like exactly 2 weeks ago.

Apparently, I'm notorious at this hospital now, as the pacemaker guy with all of the complications that never happen to anybody else. #takeyourfamewhereyoufindit (photo 7)

Me: We had to cancel our romantic bed-and-breakfast 15th anniversary getaway because of this crap. At least I do get a bed and breakfast here.

Yeah, comprehensively expensive ones. You could stay on the French Riviera for less.

Bexa: Make sure to "pace" yourself this time so this doesn't happen again, you stubborn goofus.

Deborah: You just fancy the nurses...!

Me: The guy in the photo IS my nurse.

Tina: Just think: YOU will go down in the medical field as the fella that made pacemaker implantation high risk!

7/9/17
Looks like they're keeping me in the hospital until tomorrow, just to be sure about the infection. At least the fever's gone. #justanothermagicalweekend

And here I thought the only thing infectious was my humor.

Day Two. (photo 8)

Alaena: I'm not sure last night totally counts as a day.

Me: Felt like a freaking year. #Einsteinsaystimeisrelative

Jim: When you put up those fingers knuckles out, it's rude. But you probably know that.

I did. That's why Churchill's supposed V for Victory sign was hilarious. He was flipping off the Nazis.

Me: Jeez, I look like a creepy pedophile in this picture.

Jeri: "Send me TWO children."

And here's Round 5 of the intravenous antibiotics. #neveradullmoment

Now they're giving me my 6th freaking dose of the IV bug killers, for all the good that it's doing. #probablygetkidneyfailureontopofeverythingelse.

7/10/17
Good news: the fever lasted a hot minute and went away.

Bad news: IV dose #7 started leaking at 4:25 a.m. when the line twisted inside my freaking vein. So they had to pull it and jab me in the other arm.

This will become a theme later, one that I could've lived without (or maybe not, come to think of it).

Sharon: This is a test...had it been an actual emergency you would have been given instructions.

Doctor just said that all of the blood cultures are sterile, which is good. But since he can't yet 100% rule out pacemaker lead infection inside the heart, he's sending me home for 1 or 2 weeks of daily outpatient visits to keep nuking me with Roundup or whatever they've been pouring into me, just to be sure. IV #8 currently in place.

At least I'm outta here.

M Cd: Outta there? But for how long? If I were you, I wouldn't waste time before filling out those organ donor cards. I could use a brain transplant.

Me: I have a brain the size of a planet. It wouldn't fit.

Thank you, Douglas Adams. Here's hoping you took your towel with you into the afterlife. Or après-vie.

David: Get out of there before they break out the leeches.

Sorry, naturopathic care isn't covered by my plan.

The hopefully final echocardiogram just finished. I think that makes 5 of those and 3 chest x-rays since this all started. Plus 2 pacemakers, a heart needle, 2 resuscitations, and 8 rounds of heavy-duty antibiotics. #thankgawdforschooldistrictinsurance

Scott: No partridge in a pear tree?

Does the raven perched above the door count?

Sal: I'm assuming they do NOT serve fries with any of that?!?

Shit, shit, shit, shit, shit! Not only am I not going home today, I have to get 2 IV antibiotic treatments a day, an hour each, for the next 6 fucking weeks!!!

Everybody needs to avoid me. I'm about to throw a chair through the window.

I might've, too, except the chair was too damned heavy to lift.

Hope: Wow! Do you have to be in the hospital for that or can you go in for those?

Me: Done at home. I have to do it to myself.

"Do it to myself." If you're disappointed that there's no off-color joke on that, sorry. Even I have standards. I don't pick low-hanging fruit...unless it's an eggplant emoji.

I'm Asperger's-clumsy. I can trip over a paper clip and have run face-first into my own classroom door. The doctors didn't think this through.

Cerene: Jeez, Terry! Did they go roll you on the floor before popping you open?!

Alaena: Did they find something in one of the cultures?

Me: Nada. This is totally on mere speculation and over-caution.

Johnnie: Is this the results of a life of cigarettes and whiskey and wild, wild women?

Me: It's the result of a life of moderation and spectacular physical workouts.

Judith: When I had my last hip replacement and it infected, I needed two intravenous per day for 6 weeks too. They sent me home with an IV port and some fancy little balls full of meds that were pressurized . I just hooked them up and sat for about 35 minutes while they infused. Worked great— free to do what I liked the rest of the time and did the trick. Hopefully, you can get the same. Easy-smeezy.

Janet: That sounds like what they are going to do.

Just spent a glorious hour and a half getting a long-term PICC line implanted in my upper arm and all the way into my FREAKING HEART. This just gets better and better. At least the X-ray lass was extremely photogenic.

Nope, that Y chromosome didn't go anywhere.

Rebecca: Just think, no more IV sticks as long as the PICC line is in place. BTW, all X-ray techs are easy on the eyes. That's because we keep the lights dim in the room.

Me: This one looked to be a 19-year-old student. And they brought the cart to my room.

Curbside irradiation service. Just another perk we offer here.

7/11/17
Well, 9 rounds of IV antibiotics may or may not be killing the bad
bacteria, but it's certainly nuked my intestinal microflora.
#thatwasadisgustingmess #timeforprobioticyoghurt

Cerene: Ugh. Hope you won't need a fecal transplant... that would be crappy.

That might've been a preferable transplant option, considering. It's a real thing. You have to feel for whoever has to do those all day as a career choice.

Day 4. (photo 9)

Jim: You're missing a finger? Has the accounting department been by already?

It was a friendly warning from Vinny and Sal.

Scott: I'm pretty sure that would be an arm and a leg.

Julie: Does your hospital have a points card? Maybe you can get a free procedure.

The doctor who's supposed to get me out of here said he'd be here
by 2. So, of course, it's an hour past that and no freaking sign of him.
I just reminded the hospital that I'm a patient not a prisoner and I'm
leaving regardless, so something better happen. There's probably a
cardiologists' poker game running long.

Update: And, of course, he showed up 2 nanoseconds after I
complained.

Probably 'saving a life' or some equally lame excuse.

(Janet) Unhappy about the antibiotics is an understatement. Terry is not the most cooperative of patients and will Google medical journals and websites to research thoroughly anything pertaining to his medical problems. He was not happy about having to undergo six weeks of a PICC line just on spec. I was not happy having to be the one who administered the infusions and having to nag him into sitting there quietly on the

schedule. It didn't help that his trough readings were always off and a nurse would arrive at 7am to take more blood every couple of days.

Nurses keep stopping by my room to inform me that they were on the ICU team that revived me 2 weeks ago and that I look a lot better now than on my near deathbed. It was like I was a saint receiving pilgrims.

Home again, home again, jiggety-jog.

David: No running with the IV pole...

Can't run. It's not an election year.

7/12/17
So, this is our 15th wedding anniversary. We marked the occasion by Janet learning how to hook me up to an IV bag twice a day.

Christine: That's love, right there.

Dean: Party animal.

I do know how to show a girl a good time. "That's it! Oh, yeah! Infuse me, baby! Do it!"

Married to Janet Moongoddess Smith for 15 Years. (photo 10)

Janet designed and sewed those Hollywood-caliber costumes herself (she trained at the same Manhattan fashion school as Calvin Klein). The way to a man's heart is through his trunk hose (that's the big, poofy, knee-high 'pants' that men wore back then).

Ann-Elise: You guys look so cool!

Me: Actually, we were close to heat exhaustion at that event.

7/13/17
We got married by a judge on the 12th, but then did the actual

ceremony the next day, 15 years ago, in the middle of a Shakespeare show we were in. Yes, we had the *Princess Bride* vows: "Mawwiage...that bwessed sacwament...that dweam within a dweam..." (photo 11)

Me: My best man ran me through the neck with 4 feet of Italian steel a bit earlier in the evening for a *Macbeth scene*. #respect

Immediately after the 'I do's', we sat on stage and played Theseus and Hippolyta for the Pyramus and Thisbe scene from 'A Midsummer Night's Dream' You know, like all weddings do.

7/14/17
Yesterday was the first day in over a week without any sort of fever or night sweats.

And because it was Bastille Day, I got French fireworks.

Julia: Like I say — do what the doctor tells you, until he tries to attach leeches.

Me: Not much difference between leeches and this catheter.

Janet: The leeches would do the attaching by themselves.

Me: Less work for you.

7/16/17
Setting up Janet's new computer, after about 10 years with the old dinosaur. Send sherpas, medics, and Seal Team 6.

Brian: What about lawyers, guns and money?

Couldn't hurt. We could sacrifice the lawyers on a burning pyre to Bill Gates.

No fever since Wednesday. Lung congestion/coughing nearly all

gone. Pacemaker incision nearly invisible after 3 weeks. Feeling 3/4 normal. #I'vekickedDeath'sass

Too bad Death's ass had armor plating. #myfoothurts

First bath in 8 days, what with hospitals and IV's and such. Had to wrap the catheter site in Saran Wrap and then wear a 3-foot alien condom on my arm, provided by home health care. #toosexy (photo 12)

I look like I'm about to artificially inseminate a moose.

Rebecca: Pictures or it didn't happen. Not the bath, please.

Sorry. The moose was too shy.

Nap: Welcome in the club. I've got my third one. Wished they provide a zipper for it.

Well, that turned out to be a good idea…for the cover, anyway.

'Pacemaker' is so boring. I plan to tell the curious that it's the tip of a Viking spear. #somuchcooler (Photo 13)

Eileen: I was thinking the Alien.

The term they prefer is xenomorph. Try to be 'woke', sheesh.

Adam: Scarab beetle.

Garalt: When someone tries to touch it say: "Don't touch the larvae, they have yet to pupate. They're my little friends."

Curtis: All you need is an arc reactor.

Tina: Looks like a horse bite to me…you must have been in the Wild West!

Melanie: My kid once upon a time took a header off his scooter, resulting in a broken arm. I had to educate him in the art of Epic Storytelling. "I fell off my scooter" is so... pedestrian.

7/18/17
So...the medical people just called and said that yesterday's blood tests indicate that they've been over-dosing me with the scary antibiotics to the point of potential kidney failure (!) and to skip tonight's infusion entirely. They're rushing new, lower dosages here as we speak. WTAF??? #ain'tmodernmedicinegrand?

You know, my kidneys wouldn't fail if they'd taken notes on the reading. I put it up on the board and told them in class three times!

The hospital gave me the world's lamest bong. But at least I can inhale enough to max out the gauge. #fearmylungfunction (photo 14)

Dave: It's more of a reverse bong.

Scott: Would that be a bing? And since it's lame, it must be a badder-bing.

Thank you, folks! You've been a great crowd. Scott will be here all week. Please tip your server.

7/22/17
First back-to-school classroom purchase made: a *Despicable Me* fart gun. Now I'm ready to face those urchins.

When some student gives me a wrong answer, they get a fart blast. Sometimes I even use the toy gun.

I've lost over 12 pounds since getting out of the hospital and being forced to eat literally nothing enjoyable anymore (no cream, chocolate, alcohol, carbonation, citrus, etc.). Most of that was probably water accumulation from all of the saline infusions, but still...

Those who have actually seen me will be thinking, "12 pounds from WHERE???"

Jim: Well - you always had a huge butt.

Me: Oh, please. You can literally grab my butt in one hand. That's not an invitation, BTW. #buymedinnerfirst

7/26/17
So...what's the penalty for violently shoving a pointless IV antibiotic kit up the back end of every member of the local medical profession? Asking for a friend.

Combine it with fecal feeding and charge **them.**

7/29/17
Got the pulse up to 160 on the bike (25 miles). In theory, that's 100% of maximum for my age. So I guess I'm pretty much healed, pacemaker-wise. Next weekend I'm officially off of all physical restrictions, not that I've been paying much attention to them anyway.

"Healed...I don't think that word means what you think it means."

7/30/17
Tried jogging with the pacemaker today, 5 weeks after my cyborging. 1st quarter mile felt like the Bataan Death March. 2nd quarter was only about 5 seconds slower than normal pace before all of this happened. #stillnotdeadyet

Maria: They will be assimilated. Resistance will be futile.

7/31/17
My honeybunch checked the health insurance site and apparently my first hospital visit, for the 'pacemaker with life-threatening complications', was about $80,000.

#thisiswhyeverybodyneedsinsurance

If you know any idiots who refuse to buy insurance only because 'I'm young and healthy, why waste the money?', I'm a living cautionary tale.

8/4/17
Good thing I'm able to run again. Just had to sprint 200 meters with the basset hound to get home ahead of a hellacious thunderstorm.

Me: And when I use 'sprint' and basset hound' in the same sentence, I'm aware of the irony.

8/19/17
The wretched antibiotic IV catheter has been forever removed from my arm. Woo-hoo!

Jennifer: At least it was only in your arm.

She was right. The urinary catheter experience was in my future…twice.

8/24/17

Had the appointment with the guy who put in the pacemaker 2 months ago today. He used the world's most expensive laptop to scope it and declare everything hunky-dory. I'm as 'cured' as I'm ever going to be. I don't have to see him for a year. Woo-hoo!

*He did mention that before jabbing that spear of Achilles into me and draining the pericardium, I'd been about **10 minutes from being dead**. Wasn't too forthcoming with that tidbit of info at the time.*

David: Just don't lose the warranty on that thing.

Not a good time for built-in obsolescence.

9/11/17
Upon sober reflection, perhaps running 2 miles during my plan period today after, the 30 miles of beastly bike climbing yesterday, was...unwise. #naptime

Jim: You chose... poorly...

Allusion to the end of 'Indiana Jones and the Last Crusade', choosing the real Holy Grail (the wrong choice is fatal).

Janet: Unwise should be your middle name.

Me: Unwise Gamgee.

9/27/17
Yeah, I just had to log onto a website to set the time on my watch. #fitbitproblems

And now I have an even more complicated Apple watch. But at least this one has Mickey Mouse telling me the time out loud: "It's ten o'clock. Good night, pal!"

10/14/17
We have the plumber in on a Saturday. Might need a telethon to pay for this. #sendmoney #anythinghelps

Janet: We might need one for all the medical bills the insurance is refusing to pay for. Or for the lawyer we may need to make them pay for it.

2018

1/16/18
My genius retirement plan: Opening a chain of Colorado pizza, chiropractic, and pot shops called "The Pizza Joint."

It'd be a license to print money here.

1/25/18
Yeah, I explained to my class that a good example of trochaic meter is the word 'dumbass.' You got a problem with that?

"Dumbass students make me crazy." Trochaic tetrameter.

1/31/18
Just visited the cardiologist who put in the pacemaker. He literally adjusted my timing. At least he didn't insist on a lube job, too.

Me: He had to install the 'athletic' setting, because it wasn't recognizing that I was running. It wouldn't boost the heart rate and I'd get short of breath and have to stop.

2/7/18
I really want the first shot of the new *Doctor Who* season to be Jodie Whittaker driving a red Tesla convertible that she just found floating in space.

Now was that too much to ask?

2/9/18
(written in literally 15 minutes this a.m., in class, as students complained that writing sonnets was too hard)

'My teacher said I had to write this poem,
But now my mind's a shallow, tragic blank.
So all I dream about is being home,
And how my verses always really stank.
A sonnet's not my perfect cup of tea.
I'd rather take my chances picking fights,
Or risk an alternate reality,
At least that way I might seem halfway bright.
If only God had gifted me some skills,
Like Shakespeare, Milton, Marlowe...yeah, that crowd,
I might be making hundred-dollar bills,
Instead of weeping with my head all bowed.

The only verse that really matters, rap,
Pays so much better than iambic crap.'

Yeah, Lord Byron has nothing on me.

2/28/18
Waited until I was 60 with a pacemaker to finally run Bolder Boulder in May. FYI, they think **REALLY** highly of what their event is worth.

Me: They stick you in the rear unless you have a race result from a previous year proving you can run faster than 11 minutes a mile. A roadkill slug can run faster than that. #mynewrunnername

The BolderBoulder is a nationally famous 10K citizens' race through the streets of Boulder, Colorado. 50,000 runners. Bands playing on seemingly every street corner as you go. Slip-n-Slides on the side of the road. People in costumes. Very 'Colorado.'

3/1/18
I despair for the youth of today. I just asked 3 classes (80 students total) how many had **NEVER** seen a *Star Trek* episode and nearly all of them raised their hands.

Me: Then I showed them "The Trouble with Tribbles." Problem solved. America's youth redeemed.

Dean: That ain't right.

Me: International Baccalaureate kids. That's typical, actually. Most haven't seen *Star Wars*, either.

Their parents don't want to sully their Ivy League-bound minds with lowly popular culture.

Scott: "I find your lack of Lucas disturbing."

Me: David Gerrold will be in my classes all day next Wednesday, so they'll be getting up to speed in a hurry.

FYI, he wrote that episode, in 1967. Has every science-fiction writing award you'd want, from the Hugo on down. I was gobsmacked that he agreed to come to my classes and teach. Even more so that now he's an actual friend.

Jim: Need any extra adults to help manage the class?

Me: Nice try.

Veronica: Perhaps they're not nerds.

Me: They're ALL nerds, that's what's so weird.

Me: They've ALL seen *Black Mirror,* though.

Me: This prompted a discussion of cultural mythology and why societies choose certain stories to be worth valuing. And that the gods of Homer were just X-Men.

Scott: Since the Greeks believed in apotheosis, some of their gods were indeed ex-men.

Janet: As much as I enjoy *Star Wars* and the Hero's Journey, *Star Trek* addressed issues and promoted a positive future where all races and species try to get along with each other. We have most of the gadgetry now because tech nerds watched *Star Trek* and decided to make the stuff. The *Star Trek* societal future looks like it's farther away than ever.

And now Seth McFarlane's 'The Orville' is doing what the original 'Star Trek' did.

Holy crap...my student just won the Colorado Poetry Out Loud state championship (poetry reciting) and is going to nationals in D.C.

Me: We've now won this event, the National Shakespeare Competition state championship, and 7 district writing awards during my tenure. Just sayin'...

3/3/18
We're at the first annual WhimsyCon Steampunk convention in

Denver. Presented 2 author panels already and am now prepping the ever-popular Bartitsu workshop for 2 pm. Then a reading from my novel, and my renowned 63-slide PowerPoint lecture on stuff you didn't know about Jules Verne.

Bartitsu is a real mixed martial art from around 1900. A blend of boxing, wrestling, cane fighting, savate (French kickboxing), and jiu-jitsu. We learned it from Tony Wolf's books on the subject, and later brought him in to teach us in person. Amazingly, we'd been doing it properly (and teaching others) just from the books. Bartitsu is the actual discipline Sherlock Holmes uses to throw Moriarty off of Reichenbach Falls. It's mentioned by name in the story. Tony Wolf was the guy who designed the fighting styles of the various races in the 'Lord of the Rings' movies.

Fun fact about Jules Verne: his crazy nephew shot him in the foot, permanently crippling him. But he was aiming for the groin (not a joke).

Justin: Sometimes I swear you should have your own reality TV show.

Me: And after that I could be President.

Scott: "First annual?" Prepare to be assailed by the Secret Masters of English, sir.

Me: It's the first one ever and is intended to be an annual event. Assail away, haters.

3/6/18
David Gerrold was just in our living room, loving up on the basset hounds.
Rebecca: I am so jealous.

Me: As well you should be. He's an erudite hoot.

Maria: I want to love on your basset hounds.

Let me tell you, when you take David Gerrold out to dinner, awkward silences are not a problem. He told splendid stories non-stop for an hour: about Isaac Asimov, Theodore Sturgeon, *Star Trek* ("The

Galileo Seven" was the same plot as *Flight of the Phoenix*), Harlan Ellison's house, good writing vs. bad, all sorts of yummy stuff.

That was one dinner I was more than happy to pay for.

3/11/18
2 and a half hours of curling on 5 hours of sleep. Threw 30 rocks (over 1200 lbs. of granite). Everything hurts. Nap time.

Later my inability to sweep the ice without having to stop and gasp like I was sprinting uphill was a major clue that something was wrong. Even more wrong than curling.

3/13/18
Nearly 30 of years of teaching and this comment in class was a first: "My sister makes $6000 a week as a stripper."

With a two-week vacation, that's $300,000 a year. Four times what I make teaching America's youth. Pardon me while I set fire to all of my college diplomas.

Veronica: That kind of income won't last forever, so you gotta know how to invest.

Terry W.: Terry, you missed your calling.

Yeah, I'd be quite the novelty act with these scars. 'Tragic Mike.'

Jeri: Jeebus, I'm in the wrong line of work...again!

3/17/18
Ran a nonstop 5K without any pacemaker issues. The legs, however, are another story.

3/19/18
Off to the DMV. Send thoughts and prayers...and a hostage rescue team.

3/19/18
Thus ends the last day of my youth.

Me: Well, I call it 'youth.'

Dave: Yeah...21 is a major milestone.

Me: My bathrobe is 21. I am NOT joking. Got it in 1997. #polyesterneverdies

And now my heart is 3 years younger than the robe.

3/20/18
60??? How the heck did THIS happen?

Jim: Beats me. Between appendix and heart issues and falling off bikes and so on, you've tried...

Stephany: Welcome to the club, old man.

Me: Yeah, but we're 'Colorado old', which is like 45 in Kansas.

*And I will **always** be 10 months younger than you, dear.*

Sheila: What is really 'horrible'...I see this really buff guy and think "Oh, my!" then realize — I am old enough to be his, uh, mother! Damn!

Let your cougar flag fly, Sheila.

Birthday dinner at the Himalayan Bistro (sherpa stew and saag paneer), watching the women's world curling championship from Canada on the TV above the bar (Russia beating Japan, U.S. beating Switzerland), while drinking a ginger peach margarita full of Mexican blue agave tequila and French Cointreau. #aren'tweallinternational

Don't panic. The sherpa stew was not made from real sherpas.

Garalt: You're trying too hard (unless you arrived in national costume on

the back of a yak).
Me: There WAS a huge mural of yaks there.

I have a T-shirt that says, 'Yak Yeti Yak Yeti Yak.' (say it quickly).

4/1/18
Ran 4 miles for the first time in a year, before the pacemaker went in. All well and good, but I need a 14-hour nap. #oldguyworkout

Me: On the upside, I'm now in the coveted 60-year-old race category.

In ordinary citizen races, there's a steep drop-off in entries after 60. But in Colorado, a lot of those people are still averaging 6 minutes a mile. I...don't, anymore.

Though when I was in the Army 30 years ago, I could run a mile in under 6 minutes, on hills, THIRTEEN times, with a 3-minute break in between.

4/2/18
There is now a For Sale sign in front of our house.

Little did we know how much work this was going to entail, in only 8 weeks. I don't recommend frantic rush moving. It nearly did us in. 17 days in the hospital was less miserable than packing up 20 years of stuff and then cleaning the husk.

4/10/18
Few things are more hellish than the soul-destroying tedium of patrolling a classroom as SAT proctor for 4 FREAKING HOURS. #ratherwatchatrumpspeech

*They won't let you read, grade papers, or do anything to save your mind from sensory deprivation. I **might** have snuck in some casual fiction-writing, though, under the guise of taking notes on the test-takers.*

Jim: It would be slightly more tolerable if they let you wear your gear — armor, sword, dagger, pike, helm, etc. Or cosplaying Mad Eye Moody.

I could randomly shout, "You shall not pass!"

Laura: I was in the extended time...5.5 hours by myself. Can we consider that torture?

Okay, you win. I've alerted the Hague.

4/13/18

Went to a 2-hour PERA teacher retirement meeting last night, then had dinner at Village Inn with our senior citizen discount. #walkingstereotypes

Village Inn: where the average customer age has nearly 3 digits and they just assume that you qualify for the discount. It's like Denny's, but without the cosmopolitan chic.

PERA is Colorado's Public Employee Retirement Association. They hold the keys to the kingdom of you being able to afford to sit on your couch and imagine somebody else having to deal with your little darlings. Not that I don't love them all, but 30 years is a long time. This is presuming, of course, that I'll ever be able to retire. Have to have the right insurance to pay for the transplant meds.

4/14/18

Well, we didn't buy the new house just because it has 42 in the address, but that's a plus, nonetheless.

I did say early on that there would be Douglas Adams references. Janet's addicted to him, as well as Doctor Who. Toys, shirts, autographed posters…our house looks like a geek museum. There's a 42 in our house number, phone number, and in my credit card number.

4/15/18

The local curling club had their big Learn to Curl event today (40 newbies showed up). Since I have a whole 2 days experience, I became an assistant instructor.

Me: Put my first rock dead center, so at least I appeared superficially qualified.

*FYI, it's a **lot** harder than it looks when the folks on TV, who've been playing daily* *since the age of 7, do it. They can drop the rock within an inch of where they want it. I'm happy to hit that 12-foot target at all. It's a hundred feet away and all you can see is a bluish smear. All done by feel and muscle memory, neither of which is necessarily my strong suit, the Asperger's being a clumsiness-vector.*

4/19/18
Getting paid to teach *Hamlet* all day. #mylifeisbetterthanyours

Julie: I don't know about that. I'll be watching *Hamlet* at the Globe next month.

Me: But will you be getting PAID to watch it?

Julie: Who knows? It's the day of the wedding and maybe there will be an Oprah moment.

And you get a free tragedy, and you get a free tragedy…!

Ellie: Is Hamlet more Protestant, or not so much?

Me: Pretty Catholic, actually. As was Shakespeare's family, more or less secretly. Lots of references to confessions and Purgatory.

Ellie: Thank you! Gotta discuss soon with my European History class.

Glad to be of service. I presume my tutoring check is in the mail?

Iris: Outrageous fortune.

That should be the name of a pornographic Chinese cookie company.

4/22/18
Spent the morning curling. Put most of my rocks in the rings or as guards. Waiting to see if my back hurts less than the other times I did it. #it'sarealsportpeople

Note: No, it did not hurt less. Those rocks weigh 42 lbs. But I didn't slip on the ice and fracture my skull, as Janet always predicts. I've seen a guy hit his head and bleed all over the ice.

Just managed to run 5 miles for the first time since the pacemaker went in. Dead slow (as in, a dead person would have run it faster). Bolder Boulder in 5 weeks.

Scott: The fact that you're running it at all says something, considering how dire the pacemaker drama was. Patience, Jedi.

You don't know the power of the Dork Side of the Farce.

I find my lack of pace…disturbing.

5/8/18
Moved so many boxes of books to the new house in the last week that I've lost several pounds even without having time to run or bike.

Me: The books are so heavy that the car's gas mileage has gone down.

That was just the books we kept. Even more went to the library or Goodwill. We're personally responsible for global deforestation.

5/10/18
So, of the first 4 student essays I've graded today, 2 spelled my name wrong. They've been in my class since AUGUST.
Even worse, I once had a student turn in Shirley Jackson's "The Lottery" and claim he wrote it.

5/15/18
Most Colorado thing ever: the last three digits of our new phone # are 420.

And that's as close to 420 as I'll ever get, thanks to the rejection meds.

For the uninitiated: 420 is a term that originated at a California high school in 1971, referencing an afternoon meeting time for a group of stoners. It has since been co-opted as the name for an annual April 20ᵗʰ celebration of all things weedy. And since 42 in Douglas Adams' books is the answer to Life, the Universe, and Everything…

5/17/18
The moving van will be here a week for tomorrow and that'll be it for us in this house, after 20+ years.

In the end, we spent less $ on the movers than we spent on 3 roll-off dumpsters to haul our unwanted crap away. We Marie Kondo-ed the hell out of that place.

Managed to survive running a 10K for the first time since the cardiac issues last year. Pacemaker didn't malfunction and neither did the legs. SO freaking slow. I used to be able to run the whole 6.2. miles in the time I ran 4 miles in today. In my defense, the Fitbit said I was at 17,000 steps before I started the run, and it was over 80 degrees. 15 miles of running/walking/cleaning out garages & moving stuff to the new house.

Me: Anyway, Bolder Boulder is in 10 days and, apparently, I'll be able to at least plod to the end of it.

And plod was most definitely the appropriate term, though stagger, stumble, and crawl were in the, um, running.

5/25/18
Well, we've been officially moved into this new house for 3 hours ('officially' means the dogs are here). The bassets keep wondering when we're getting back in the car to go 'home.'

(Janet) Let me tell you, moving is horrible! I worked every day for over a month, sorting, boxing, dumping and giving away tons of our stuff, including most of the costumes and props. All the while contractors and assorted people were in and out of our house. Many times, I would have to drop everything and take the dogs down to my friend Michele's house and hang out while they were working. At the same time, my blood pressure was really high (what a surprise) and my doctor put me on meds which completely messed up my eyesight. I got new glasses, but the many med changes in the next year were a constant eyesight problem.

Me: 90F on the first day and, of course, the central air conditioning died.

Kelly: Pics, please, of new house.

Me: Not until we put everything away...so maybe October.

5/27/18
Got a literal spam call today, advising us of a recall on Spam.

Can't make this shit up.

5/27/18
Running the BolderBoulder tomorrow (just me and 50,000 support staff). I was amazed to notice that when I was 30, my 10K time would have had me in the top .05%. #thosedaysareSOgone #usedtorunitunder37:00

Yeah, in the late 80's, when I was an infantry officer in the Army, I was a major badass. Nobody ever believes that. Hell, they can't believe I was ever in the Army at all. Me having an Airborne badge really blows their minds.

Me: Since I didn't have a recent 10K time, they stuck me in the 36th wave with the mommies running 11:30/mile. Amazingly, there are still 60 waves behind me. #that'salotoffreakingrunners

Me: Shouldn't complain, since the whole point is to be happy that I can run it at all, instead of being, well, dead.
#pacemakerusedtomeansomethingelsewhenrunning

5/28/18
Proof of my up-before-dawn insanity today. The wife had to drive me to the bus. She seemed thrilled.

I wore a shirt that said on the back, "I may be old, slow, and have a pacemaker, but I'm still ahead of you." I now have a heart transplant version of it.

5/28/18
Well, I'm on the bus to BolderBoulder at 6:25 a.-freaking-m.

Everybody on the bus had 3% body fat and a $500 runner's watch.

5/28/18
It's awfully liberating to be running the BolderBoulder, not caring at all what my time will be. Just jogging this sucker in honor of being able to run at all.

Me: SO freaking humid. Barely staggered into the stadium at the end.

In Colorado, it's too humid to us at about 24%. We went back to my mom's house in Illinois in 2015 and nearly suffocated. Both of us have been living high and dry for too long to ever live in a humid zone again.

5/29/18
20 years ago today I got picked up at the Denver airport by a lovely lady of dubious judgment who'd agreed to let me move in with her from Texas SIGHT UNSEEN after a very few months of postal correspondence. She took me (and my basset hound) with a smile and has refrained from smothering me in my sleep ever since. #sainthood

Me: It's either the most romantic or most insane thing ever, depending on your outlook.
Oh, why do we have to choose?

Me: She literally picked me out of a catalog...because of the dog. #notjoking #mailorderhusband

That'll teach her to fall in love with basset hounds on TV without ever having been a slave to one. They're all service dogs: you spend every waking hour giving them service.

Alaena: At the time, insane was certainly my thought. But I'm glad you are here. Happy Anniversary.

Janet: And I had to drive him back to the airport the next day because he left his glasses in the rental car in Texas and they had to fly them here. All he had was his prescription sunglasses. I still let him stay. Menopausal brain does weird things.

5/21/18
BolderBoulder results: not awful, considering I merely jogged it on almost no real training (ran a 10K all of twice in the 2 weeks before the race). Good ad for the mighty Boston Scientific pacemaker corporation. Top 1/4 in my age group, top 1/3 of all men, top 1/4 of all runners. 38,000 people finished behind me. (photo 15)

Me: The Kenyan guy that won the whole thing ran it 33 minutes faster than me. In my best shape ever, 30 years ago, he still would've beaten me by over a mile. But I would've been 200th place out of 50,000.

For those wondering why the Kenyans always kick ass in distance running: Nairobi is 7500 feet above sea level, so they have extremely efficient lungs. Plus, hungry lions are really, really fast.

6/10/18
Jeez. I'm living in a community with annoying rules, fertilizing my lawn because it isn't green enough, programming my irritation system, and going to block parties. Everything I swore I'd never do. #justkillmenow #sothesearetheendtimes

Me: At least we removed the Jesus plaque on the lawn and dropped an enormous Buddha on the spot.

Alaena: Programming your irritation system eh?

Me: Well, I WAS present when the guy next door did it for me.

7/7/18
So, it would seem that if the day is going to be 100F, then 8 a.m. is already too late to start running your 5K.

Lottie: Hmm. With heart conditions? I wish you wouldn't.

Me: The 10K in Boulder in May was much hotter at that time of day, and uphill. The uphill 5K's on the bike at 14% grade are a harder slog. (it's a REALLY good pacemaker).

I had bradycardia, abnormally low heartbeat. Once I got moving and keep moving, the pacemaker wasn't needed and would just stay dormant. But as soon as I stopped, the pulse would try to drop from 160 to 0 in two minutes. Then the wonder-toy would kick in to maintain 50 BPM, barely enough to keep me awake.

7/9/18
So...David Gerrold just drove up to our house and bought us brunch at a French bistro. #notyourusualMonday

It seems he's addicted to sage derby cheese, which is as green as an algae-covered pond. I shouldn't talk, I put dill pickles on my peanut butter sandwich.

7/12/18
16 years of wedded bliss today. That's MY opinion, anyway. Janet's mileage may vary.

This isn't counting the 4 years of joyous shacking up before actually putting a ring on it.

7/12/18
Spent our anniversary buying a new refrigerator. #theromanceneverdies

Mark: Proof that your romance hasn't "cooled."

Me: You need to chill out (icy glare).

Jim: Trying to impress 'er with a new compressor.

Tina: Ouch, they're getting worse!

Tina: The romance gave me cold chills.

Maria: You sentimental fool.

Gonna please her with a freezer.

7/31/18
We have our tickets for full-contact armored jousting at the Boulder County Fair next Tuesday night. Do you?

Mandy: Full-contact armoured jousting — a.k.a. breaking limbs being pushed off a horse at a gallop wearing tin cans. I am, of course, assuming they're using blunts and not sharps.

Maria: Are you participating?

Me: The pacemaker means my days of full contact anything are over for good.

Plus, the smallest guy was about 6' 4" and 240 lbs. And he still looked like chopped sausage at the end (the **winner** *had to be helped off the field). I'm currently 5'11" and 155 lbs. Their empty armor outweighs me. I couldn't even stand up in that stuff.*

Maria: Dang...because...I would totally watch that.

I'm now over 10 pounds lighter, thanks to my Extended Hospitalization Diet Plan™.

8/4/18
43 miles on the bike. Didn't thoroughly check the local race route, so I can now honestly say that I have (accidentally and briefly) ridden in the Ironman Triathlon. #sothat'swhytheywereapplaudingme.

Me: 95 degrees.

Maria: Showoff!

Really happy they didn't make me ride the whole 100+ miles. My butt wasn't prepped for that.

8/22/18
The new kids all come in for the first day of class and segregate

themselves, boys on one side and girls on the other. Weird.

Jim: Time to show the wedding dance scene from *Fiddler on the Roof*.

They do it every year, so it must be... ♫ Traditiionnn!"

M Cid: You should sort them by how much you like them individually (and exclaiming the fact) and the only way they can move out of their seat is by challenging the next seat to a duel.

Me: Much like I do my FB friends.

9/2/18
Well, my record of 7 years without a serious bike wreck lasted all of 4.7 miles today. Broke a pedal clip on my bike shoe and got overbalanced. Almost saved it by getting low across the top bar, but no. A Superman flying leap fully on top of the bike. Every limb bleeding, chest impact just missed the pacemaker, and upper groin impact (!). No head contact, though. Looks like 7 wounds/bruises. Waiting for Janet to rescue me. Luckily, this was on the bike path and not in the middle of Labor Day traffic. And people were near to pick me up. No actual ambulance needed, unlike 2011.

The bike, though, will need surgery. Rear derailleur trashed, handlebars and brake lever bent, handlebar tape shredded. Might be other problems. Not sure yet. Probably need new bike shoes. These may be too old to securely hold onto the pedals.

And I shredded my fancy-shmancy new gloves.
#ouch #I'vehadbetterlongweekends

Einstein was right: time is relative. He said if you're with your beloved, 2 hours seems like 2 seconds. If you put your hand on a hot stove, 2 seconds seems like 2 hours. I had a lot of time to contemplate the suckiness of my situation during that 2 hours on my way to the ground.

Fun fact: If I hadn't survived the 2011 wreck, my last word on earth then would've been, "Shiiiit!"

The groin (over the left femoral artery) turned blacker than licorice and was the most horrifying thing about the whole experience.

Eileen: This ER nurse cannot tell you how relieved she is that you weren't on the road at the time. Cars just never get the fact that bike (motorized or not) crashes take a hella less time to happen, so the car can't stop in time. Sorry about the all-over road rash. Since you've done this before, I know you know you'll be sore tomorrow. Ice, ice, baby. Speaking of babies, baby yourself.

Despite Colorado being Cycling Central of America, there's a lot of obnoxious driver animosity toward bikes. People have been run over on purpose by asshats who think only their unmuffled pickup truck should be on the road. That said, a car next to the bike path screeched to a halt when I went down and offered assistance. Another time, years ago, when I blew a tire on a dirt curve and went down, a total stranger threw me and the bike in his truck and drove me home.

Another fun fact: cars can stop quicker at 20 mph than bikes can.

Janet: Looks like mostly scrapes and a few bruises. Head and helmet are fine. Elbows and knees are scraped like when we were kids and fell on roller skates. He was 5 minutes from the house on the bike path, thankfully.

Me: Luckily there's a full bottle of 94-proof Tanqueray gin in the house.

Dave: I keep thinking how Don Armado became the Phantom of the Opera. I hate that this shit happens to you. Honestly, on the karma front busting your hand and losing a third of your face should have evened up the score.

He's referring to the 2011 wreck, where I had no skin on the entire left side of my face and a broken right pinkie finger; this was less than a week before I had to play Don Armado in Shakespeare's 'Love's Labour's Lost.' Thankfully, I'm a very quick healer and the face damage could be covered by makeup come showtime. The finger had a splint on it and I covered it with a foppish handkerchief. My swordfight was a nervous, careful affair. Didn't help that most shows were outdoors in a 104-degree heat wave. Oh, yeah…I wore real steel armor, too.

Fiona: Owwww! Apply internal alcohol rub and a hot bath!

Francine: Glad you can talk about it from home and not a hospital. Be gentle with yourself as your body heals. And, I hope you feel better soon.{gentle hugs}

Scott: Losing a pedal is a terrifying thing — been there twice, though with somewhat less extensive results. Hope you feel better soon.

Liana: Maybe it's time for a stationary model.

*No faster than I go, it **is** a stationary model.*

Maria: You need to stop this shit. It's not a competition who can get the most accidents in the most fanciful manner possible.

No, it's a competition for the most exotic and weird medical crap. I'm lapping the field.

9/4/18
So, the upside of Sunday's nasty bike wreck: my $1000 of clothes, Fitbit, bike computer, and helmet are undamaged (not to mention the hellishly expensive cardiac pacemaker), unlike my 60-year-old body.

Me: Can't say the same for the bike, though. Luckily, most of what has to be replaced was about to wear out anyway.
#notthepreferredmethodforgettingatuneup

Maria: You have a bike computer?

Me: Sits on the handlebars. GPS calculates where you are, how fast, altitude, temperature, all that stuff, and then you download it. Way cool.

Now if they'd only install a gyroscope to keep me upright...

Cindi: Wow, Terry I am so sorry to hear that you had another bike wreck! But I am very glad that you are not hurt as badly as before. I recently wrecked my bike and had bruises for weeks, not to mention a bruised ego for having wiped out in front of several people! I get it about the 60-year-old body! Ice, rest and Advil should be your friends right now! Also happy your technology made it through unscathed. Take care of yourself!

Johnnie: Good luck with the recuperating, Terry. Remember when we were kids and fell off of them daily without a scratch.

No, but I remember my dad shoving my 4 or 5-year-old self down the street and watching me crash in a bloody heap. Then he jammed me back on and did it again and again, thinking I was going to magically 'get it.' All I got were innumerable bloody wounds and a lifetime of resentment. Later, I did magically get it, when he wasn't there to watch. Great times for enlightened parenting, the mid 60's.

9/26/18
According to the cardiologist last week, when they 'adjusted my timing' in February (pacemaker), the thing was making my heart beat only 9% of the time. Now it's keeping me going 84% of the time. It still drops down to 49 BPM if I sit for more than 2 minutes. #butthebatterywilllastforanother15years?

It was the annual checkup, plus I was feeling weird tinglies in my chest, down my arms, and up into my throat. He immediately scheduled a treadmill stress test, 'just to be on the safe side.' It turned out to be a strange new meaning of 'safe' that I wasn't previously aware of (thanks again to Douglas Adams).

9/27/18
Cardiac stress test today at the hospital (yay). I ran longer than the average for my age (not unusual) and apparently have nothing clogged, just the wonky electrical system that the pacemaker fixed (yay again, with more feeling). Not unexpected, since I didn't have a heart attack running the Bolder Boulder in May (10K).

Guess they should have a mechanic look at that expensive stress machine, huh? Is it still under warranty?

David: Last time a doctor told me to take a stress test, I said, "I don't need a stress test. I raised a teenager."

Me: I raised several thousand, one classroom at a time.

David: I bow to your expertise.

Me: It's still not the same as actually raising even one 24/7, alone. You win the crown.

Rebecca: Try teaching college, they think they know everything.

David: I have taught college. <shudder>

Rebecca: I am now retired, do not miss the arguing. I felt like I should have 'Read the Syllabus' tattooed on my forehead.

Me: I've taught those little darlings, too. (eye roll)

12/7/18
An injection in each arm and a blood draw. That's how MY weekend started.

Dave: Oh, no...were you admitted?

Me: Just a flu shot and tetanus shot, and a blood draw to check thyroid levels.

Dave: Oh, phew! I don't want you anywhere near a hospital for a long time. Like at least another 40 years.

It turned out to be a lot less than 40 years…67 days, in fact.

Jonathan: For a second, I thought it might be vibranium implants.

The magical wonder-metal in the Black Panther movie. Captain America's shield is mostly made of it. Though Jonathan might've meant adamantium, which formulates Wolverine's skeleton and claws. #toogeekytolive

Me: Oh, I already have those. #fearme

Yes, Amazon's splendid algorithm just sent me an email suggesting that I buy a book I actually wrote.

Good as 'Brimstone and Lily' is, in my minimally humble opinion (hey, it won an award *or two), I have more than enough copies without paying myself a $2 royalty by spending $19.*

Scott: Well, they know what suits you. It's as if the author knew the contents of your head!

Shaindel: They do that to me DAILY. It would increase my book sales.

Cathryn: But they won't let you review it...so unfair.

2019

1/18/19
♫ **"Hello, Wellbutrin, my new friend..."**

Eric: ♫ "I come to be mellow with you again..."

Me: Had a meltdown 5 minutes before taking the first one, so clearly, I need it.

Some mild depression comes with the mild autism. In me it manifests in out-of-control, furniture-breaking rages over nothing. Those have significantly decreased with the med and have disappeared completely with the new heart. That's good, because Janet and the hound don't like hiding in another room, waiting for the Tasmanian Devil to go away. No fun for me, either, as they feel like the seizures that they essentially are.

(Janet) Not disappeared entirely. There still are episodes of prickliness ,especially when driving, but not quite as bad as they were. The Prednisone can cause anxiety as well as the hands shaking.

To access the photos/videos/links:
www.terrykroenungink.com/246-2/

2) BLISSFULLY UNAWARE

February 13-March 30, 2019

So…according to Mensa, the international intelligence organization, I have an IQ in the 98ᵗʰ or 99ᵗʰ percentile, depending on which test you go by (that and $4.50 will get you a latte at Starbucks). This towering intellect enabled me to instantly realize that the symptoms I experienced from September 2018 on were clearly cardiac in origin, and I naturally rushed to my doctor to —

Oh, who are we fooling? My 145+ brain remained utterly clueless and I just kept on hoping that the chest pains and shortness of breath were merely indigestion, weak physical conditioning, some dietary glitch, demonic possession…anything but heart stuff. It's a wonder that I lived to type this.

This would be a good place for a shout-out to Longs Peak Hospital in Longmont, practically next door to our house, for their stellar diagnostic/emergency care during my 2 ER visits. It's thanks to you that I made it to Anschutz at all. In fact, I'm shocked, SHOCKED! (quite literally).

During the time of Part 2, early 2019, I was walking the halls during my planning periods, the weather usually being so crappy that exercising outside could involve light-sabering your poor dead tauntaun and crawling inside for warmth. Teachers and students would often ask me if I was okay, which is what we call a 'freaking clue' in the heart biz.

After the first ER visit, that gloriously ironic Valentine's Day heartisode, the comments and questions increased, as did the symptoms. At least now I had some idea what was wrong and how bad it was likely to get, as I clung to a brick wall in the corridor with my head spinning, sucking wind. That idea grew exponentially in March, as I was run through every heart test known to man, from echocardiograms to nuclear PYP scans. The only thing they didn't do was have Ant-Man shrink down and swim into my ventricles to take selfies. Too bad, because that would've cleared up a whole lot of confused diagnoses.

2/13/19
Well, this wasn't the plan for today. (photo 16)

Update: they saw an elevated cardiac protein (Troponin) result in the blood test that usually indicates something less than great. So I get to spend Valentine's Day in a #@%! hospital room.

I've been running and biking like a fiend for 50 years to avoid this crap. Not happy.

Me: Admit it, you envy my sexy old-guy lifestyle. FYI, this is mostly an abundance-of-caution visit due to intermittent shortness of breath with no obvious cause and weird chest pains that I'm hoping are just reflux-related.

Man, was I a clueless moron at that stage. Google exists for a reason, dude.

David: The things that some people will do to get out of running the marathon.

Me: It got me out of a faculty meeting, actually.

Not a joke. I'd been feeling these symptoms off and on for 2-3 months and did the logical man-thing: I ignored them. But that day was the second Wednesday of the month and there was a faculty meeting after school. I'm not a fan of big crowded rooms that I don't have control of. Not in a good mood anyway, due to the symptoms (the chest pains had become significant and frequent, along with shortness of breath that made me stop walking in the school hall), so I sent myself to the ER just as school ended. A damned good thing I did, too.

Me: 4 hours and they still haven't moved me from the ER to a real room.

Janet: What's up with that? They have a room for you and just need to clean it. I would tell them that they had better get you something to eat or you will be even crankier.

Probably removing the body and spraying some Lysol and air freshener.

Jim: Don't be one of those health nuts lying in bed dying of nothing.

Hey, I keep trying to kill myself on the public thoroughfares. Is it my fault that I have a vibranium skeleton?

2/14/19

In theory I had 8 hours of sleep. In actuality they woke me at 1 a.m. for some random questions, at 2 a.m. to take blood (5 of those so far), and the IV alarm went off 4 times, claiming that the line was blocked (it wasn't). Not giving this hyper-expensive B &B a great Yelp review.

It's not lost on me that I was in for a heart issue on Valentine's Day. Good thing it wasn't Halloween.

Me: Plus the 45-minute echocardiogram at 7-flipping-a.m.

Me: At least I have a hot blonde cardiologist here.

Hi, Dr. Carlyle! Take that in the spirit it was intended. If it weren't for your competence, you'd be billing one less patient these days. Thanks.

Russell: We're all with you, Terry. Not literally, of course; that would be weird. And probably expensive. But we are with you.

Too bad. We could all split the bill.

1 meal in the past 48 hours. Somebody at this hospital needs to make a decision on whether their exploratory procedure is happening or not, so I can wallow in the splendor of their cuisine.

'Wallow' being the operative word, as it's not quite 'swallow.'

Marti: Do not, I repeat, do not order any jello!

You know I did. The green stuff, if memory serves.

Me: So once again, I can't have a 'normal' cardiac issue.

No blockage, everything's working fine, but my heart walls are extra-thick, which reduces the volume it pumps. It may just be athlete's heart, caused by years of running and biking. That's fixable by going cold turkey on big exercise for a few months. But it may also be some exotic disease layering deposits inside the heart, which is way more problematic. But they still don't know why I get short of breath walking and not running.

No one has ever figured that out, to this day. Maybe just simple momentum. I should consult Dr. Newton.

Cynthia: So, just run everywhere. Run from the living room to the dinner table, from the car to the house, etc.

That's literally what they made us do at Officer Candidate School at Ft. Benning.

Me: It may also be the cause of my needing a pacemaker at an unusually 'young' age.

Now they're pretty much dead certain of that.

Home again. Out of the hospital and home. Less than 24 hours, a personal record. Walked around the unit 3 times, both before and after lunch, even climbed stairs, trying to make the symptoms return. Nothing before lunch, only a tiny brief bit after. Might simply be a full stomach constricting the already-constricted left ventricle. Tests due back in a week or two. Who knows?

Liana: Good news that it appears to be nothing dire.

Me: I wish that were true, having seen the test results.

2/16/19
Yes, I just got an Apple Watch 4. No, I don't know how to work it

yet.

I got the pricey thing because if you fall down and don't move for a minute, it asks if you're okay. If it gets no response, it calls 911 for you and directs the EMT's via GPS. One wonders if there's a birth coach version. It does have an app that occasionally tells you to breathe.

And 4 ½ months later I still don't know how to work all of it.

One really shouldn't read one's cardiac tests in detail and then dwell on them. I just checked to see if my insurance covered heart transplants.

In short order I learned all the cool cardio-lingo, thanks to Googling every third word in abstruse medical journals. 'Sarcoidosis is a multisystem, granulomatous disease of unknown etiology.'

Me: This'll drive you nuts.

Me: Doesn't look great, though.

Amarinda: They can do amazing stuff now. Like Steve Austin. They'll make you better than you were before.

And charge about the same $6 million as the TV show, too.

I'm not insensible to the irony of being completely exhausted by just bringing the new elliptical machine into the house.

Me: In my defense, I'm nearly 61 and my heart has gone over to the enemy.

Me: Sucker weighs 300 pounds (the elliptical, not my heart).

Though when they eventually yanked it out and weighed the enlarged monstrosity, it wasn't short of that by much.

Curtis: When you say, "It is with a heavy heart," you're not kidding.

Janet: Putting the darn machine together may finish both of us off.

Me: All done, and we're still married.

2/19/19
8 months ago I ran Bolder Boulder. 4 months ago I biked up a 13% hill. Now I can't run more than 150 steps without stopping to gasp for air. This heart thing is progressing at a scary rate.

Me: When I mentioned heart transplants the other day, I wasn't joking, alas. The cardiologist said it was a possibility if all else fails. Apparently, I have some sort of genetic curse and all my decades of healthy living were of no help.

No cardiac history in the family, either. Well, there is now.

Me: On the upside, I have no blockages anywhere, so it wasn't a total loss. The clean living accomplished **something**.

Maria: Yikes, man, that IS scary. Keep us posted. The good news is — this is, after all, 21st century. We can rebuild you. We have the technology.

So, what's the record for '$6 Million Man' allusions?

Me: Except to rebuild this, somebody else had to be dead.

That is the downside to all of this. Good thing I'm already on anti-depressants.

Dustin: What's wrong with you, Uncle Terry?

Leti: Hypertrophic cardiomyopathy.

A catch-all term when they don't actually know what the cause is. Abnormal thickening of the heart muscle. Causes heart failure.

Referred to a specialist in heart failure and transplant. That's a great start to my week.

Me: Hopefully, he'll come up with some genius workaround.

Becky: Saw you walking rounds at school today. Feeling better?

Me: Comes and goes.

Scott: I have a buddy who had a transplant...he is as right as rain, and if you need to get one, you will be, too...I just know it.

2/20/19
Normal walk in the hallway just now. After about 500 steps I was out of breath, chest pain, and had to stop. Swanky Apple watch says my pulse got up to 150. That's about 95% of my maximum. That used to be my racing pulse. #screw this

Me: Why does this only happen at school????

That was the weird thing. It very rarely hit anyplace else but school

Jim: Could be environmental. Could be you've developed an allergy to work.

Me: I've had said allergy for 60 years.

They were extensively renovating our school at the time. For a while I foolishly hoped that it was a reaction to something in the construction dust. I did a lot of foolish hoping.

2/21/19
I have a cardiology appointment every Monday in March. #funtimes

Me: Just one non-stop party. That will bring the various doctor visits since the school year started to about 15.

Me: On March 4 I get to be radioactive.

Like Chernobyl-level glow-in-the-dark radioactive, as it turned out. You could've cooked your lunch with me.

Getting dubious about the accuracy of this Apple Watch. It just claimed my pulse was 207.

Later I found out that it gave the same readings, within a single beat, as the Cardiac ICU monitor that had 10 leads attached to me. I could've left the watch on and endured a lot less annoyance. Plus, the ICU machine didn't say "Good morning, pal!" in Mickey Mouse's perky little voice.

2/22/19
Radioactive technetium-99m stannous pyrophosphate (PYP). This test looks to be an unfettered joy on March 4.

Alaena: You know, if you stayed off Google you might be a happier person.

Janet: I second that suggestion! My blood pressure meds have been doubled as it is and it may not be enough.

Me: Knowledge is power, ladies.

Knowledge is also freaking terrifying, as students of proctology will attest.

4 chest pain episodes and 26 shortness-of-breath events since Tuesday morning.

Me: Thus the extreme concern in the local medical community.

Julia: Are you at the doctor?

Me: No, they sent me home and scheduled a ton of tests for early March. I've already had over 2 dozen.

Deborah: Have they considered an inflammation of the ribs? It's called costocondritis. People come down with this after an illness with a bad cough. Hard to diagnose.

Me: I definitely have a heart issue. The left ventricle is all messed-up.

Garalt: Wow, Terry, this isn't getting simpler, is it? I'm hoping they locate the blockage and unblock it so you can again do the Bard justice.

Me: There's no blockage, though. My plumbing is crystal-clear. That's the mystery. May be a nasty genetic thing that's making the left ventricle thicken and stiffen, thus less efficient. It's the speed of the progression that's worrisome.

2/23/19
Looks like my acting days are over. I can't even get through half of "Now are the days of our discontent..." without stopping to gasp for breath. In 2012 I played King-freaking-Lear. Less than 3 months ago, I did extended speeches and scenes at our Shakeshop.

Julie: Terry, my dear old friend. Stop the self-torment. It may take time, but you will be back to what you lost. I have faith in your determination.

Maria: They are not over. You are just on health leave. We are all rooting for you.

Cindi: Baby steps right now. You are a very strong determined man. Just give yourself time and keep practicing your breathing. At least you still have your memory, unlike some people our age. Being fit up until this happened has probably served you well either by delaying the onset or the severity of your condition. You are entitled to time to grieve due to the changes you are facing. Give yourself time to do so. Self-care is important at this time! And remember you have many friends and past students who are all pulling for you and sending positive energy your way.

Jim: Now you get to sit while torturing sword fighters.

Normally I teach stage combat on my feet, demonstrating every technique. Once the pacemaker went in, I mostly had to let Josh do that while I supervised, because an accidental sword shot to the device would've been...unfortunate.

2/26/19
Auditioning new hearts. #leaveyourresumewe'llbeintouch

They should have a Tinder app for hearts. "Hmm...too much arrhythmia...swipe left."

3/1/19
This is the sort of light reading I get to do now: "B-Type Natriuretic Peptides and Echocardiographic Measures of Cardiac Structure and Function."

Peter: The sequel was better.

Maria: Is it better than the movie?

Me: If by movie you mean my echocardiogram, the movie was a literal horror show.

(Janet) One of the joys of living with an Aspie teacher/writer is that they research everything thoroughly and feel compelled to share the info, even while I'm trying to read in bed before going to sleep. I really don't want to know every medical nuance. I have a squeamish tummy.

3/4/19
Nuclear heart test today. Here's hoping that I get bitten by a radioactive spider. That'll solve all of my health problems.

Maria: As someone who's had exposure to radiation and now has mutations to prove it, I hate to tell you, but it's nowhere near as glamorous as the comic books lead you to believe.

Maria is actually unluckier than me. She grew up near Chernobyl. Seriously.

Me: After all of the CAT scans and X-rays, I probably glow in the dark.

Jacqueline: Good luck with the test!

Me: I've been studying hard.
Should've smuggled crib notes into my right atrium.

My cardiac weirdness continues: nuclear heart test didn't work.

The radioactive goo didn't absorb into the tissues like it was supposed to. They said they'd NEVER seen that.

So after driving to Denver, staying the night in a hotel, getting a substitute teacher for the day, and taking 3 1/2 hours for the test, I have to drive into Denver during rush hour (another sub) and freaking redo it Thursday. They say they may have to do the test TWICE that day.

Then I get to go back next Monday (yet another sub) for yet ANOTHER cardio appointment so the doctor can hopefully tell me what's up with this wretched ticker.

They ended up doing it three times in all. The head transplant doctor said he'd never heard of that happening before, especially to get the wrong result.

Maria: Geez, can't they just ship you off to Chernobyl, get you radioactively saturated, and then do the damn thing?

Not after you undersold the experience by talking about your own mutations from it.

3/6/19
According to my heart log: in the past 3 weeks, 83 shortness-of-breath episodes and 17 chest pain events. #arewehavingfunyet?

Me: On the upside, I'm still my usual charming, socially adept self.

3/7/19
90-minute drive to the hospital (should've been half that). Denver gridlock everywhere (ice and fog). Nearly gave myself a stroke getting to my cardiac test. That would've been funny (sort of).

Janet: I was watching the traffic report as you were driving and it was a nightmare no matter which way you went. Fog and frozen fog on slippery roads with lots of accidents. Glad you got there and fingers crossed that it works the first time. Still foggy and frosty up here so hopefully, it will clear up by the time you come home.

Maria: They owe you a free airlift.

True. I do tend to 'drone' on.

It's a tad disturbing that the nurse just told me that I'm radioactive enough to set off their detectors in the ER and make security come running. This is the fiendish device that did it. (photo 17)

It's more than a little disturbing that they feel a need for radiation detectors in their Emergency Room. Are they expecting Spiderman? The Fantastic Four? The Hulk?

Scott: So when does the wallcrawling and webshooting start?

Serge: Remember Bruce Banner?

Me: "Teacher SMASH!"

Maria: If that doesn't make them do homework, I don't know what will.

Sarah: My grandma had a nuclear stress test done the week before they went to Costa Rica. TSA was pretty sure they had the first granny terrorist.

Sean: I got a brain scan in Denver and was given a letter to show TSA if I set off their sensors.

Should've just claimed you were a supervillain and given them an evil glare.

Sure enough, they had to give me TWO freaking nuclear heart tests back to back. 4 glorious hours of hospital frenzy. An hour of holding both arms over my head. You are now allowed to express your full-throated envy.

Janet: The nuclear goo didn't circulate through Terry like it was supposed to, which meant two trips down to Anshutz in Aurora. Monday was okay, because we stayed at the hotel across the street. They called right after we got home and rescheduled for today. The traffic was a nightmare and took double the usual time. We have to go down again on Monday to see the doctor who hopefully can figure something out. Next step might be a biopsy.

Mark: And I thought Camelot was a silly place.

Mark's really into Monty Python. It's his holy grail, his meaning of life…

Janet: And, as usual for Terry, they said, "This NEVER happens!"

Kelly: Dad called it the Kroenung curse.

Maria: Hey, you beat out US military — they spaced their nuclear tests out by a few days.

I'm da bomb, baby.

Well, the nuclear test finally worked, though I'd rather it hadn't. Cardiac transthyretin amyloidosis (ATTR). Protein deposits in the heart, constantly increasing. Weakens it. Basically, acquired heart failure, despite all of my running and biking.

Rare. Incurable. Fatal.

Kids, THIS is why you should always study for your tests. I didn't crack a book and see what happened?

Me: Laugh/cry. The only choices. You all know which one I'm picking. Let the black humor commence!

Maria: Can I do both? I am doing both.

Theresa: Well, in the words of the Monty python boys: "I'm not dead yet!"

Me: True. And I now get to up my pain-in-the-ass game. What are y'all gonna do, shoot me?
Me: Lot of leverage with the students and principals now. "Do your homework! I'm a dying man!" And I can be way late grading it, because...you know.

I actually did say this to some classes. You should've seen the look on their faces.

Beth: You'll find a way to deal with this with humor and farce, I'm sure!

Me: Hey, nobody gets out of here alive. I just get a warning, is all.

Beats tripping over your dog in the dark and choking on a spoonful of frosting.

Julie: Heart transplant?

Me: Maybe. Depends on the precise type. Could also mean a liver transplant first (the nasty proteins are made there). Nothing like a $2 million dollar surgical bill to get revenge on the insurance company.

Maria: I wish I could give you half of my liver. Unfortunately, because I've been zapped by Chernobyl, I am permanently disqualified from donating organs.

Hey, it still likely works better than mine.

Stacy: You can have half of my liver if you need it. Seriously. If we're a match, it's yours. After everything you did for us Acton kids, maybe John Acton and I could make a super hybrid mega liver, and you could have that.

FYI, that's exactly what you'd think Stacy would do (former student).

Though I'm not sure that her brother knows that he got volunteered as a liver donor. But he did donate his eyes when he played Gloucester for me in 'King Lear', so he has experience in these matters.

Giselle: Did they tell you whether it was wild type or variant?

Me: They have to do a biopsy for that. Not scheduled yet. I have an appointment with the big regional guru Monday.

Kelly: Need to call mom!

Me: Yeah, that'll be a fun time.

Geoffrey: Dude. You have all my best fucking thoughts. Live every day and get a sword in your hand and fight that death fucker off.

Geoff's my Denver stage combat instructor, going back 20 years. I did challenge Death to a sword duel, but as an aristocrat, the bastard sent a professional blade man in his place. SOB sliced my heart out.

Me: I need a triple-waving plume.

*That's an allusion to Cyrano de Bergerac. But I don't have to tell **you** that.*

Maria: I've had two whiskies and it just occurred to me: people often do prayer vigils for someone's healing, but I get a feeling that won't work for you. Do you suppose we could belly-dance you back to health?

Only if you all do it in my hospital room.

Russell: Bit of a bugger, I'd say. Are you going to keep working? You always sound as though you love it so much; so that may, in fact be a help.

Me: No choice. I need the health insurance, this being the USA and all.

Russell: F#@k.

Kubler-Ross is full of crap: 'Denial and isolation, anger, bargaining, depression, and acceptance?" Weirdly, I seem to have skipped to the last one immediately.

Julie: You never could follow directions.

So…who has a heart they aren't using?

Taryn: I would give you mine, but it died, along with my soul, some years back.

Shannon: I'd give you half my liver but it's pickled.

What about the other half?

Stephanie: As so many people these days are 'heartless,' I'm sure there are quite a few hearts to spare!

Maria: Mine is radioactive.

Perfect! So is the rest of me now.

3/8/19
This is weirdly appropriate: Apparently, I just got diagnosed during Amyloidosis Awareness Month.

Garalt: So.....according to this page you're not actually a mutant. That's awful, just awful.

He's referring to inherited amyloidosis, which is called the mutant type.

Oh, I assure you I'm still a mutant. Just not an amyloid one.

Michael: Maybe you could have chosen a less dramatic way to increase awareness.

Me: I'm dying for attention.

3/9/19
I see that my less-than-24-hours hospital stay 3 weeks ago cost the usual $30,000.

Andrea: I'm guessing this is standard now. Of course, all the physicians bill separately.

Me: I don't know who half of those people even were or what they did.

Maria: Sheesh, they ought to come with a full spa service, a personal masseuse, and a box of cigars rolled between the thighs of Balinese maidens.

If I light up a stogie and blow up the hospital's oxygen system, do I have to reimburse them?

This wretched allergy attack is so awful, I'd rather have the heart failure symptoms. #onlyjokingalittlebit

Good thing I didn't have all of that sneezing with the sawn-through sternum. Ouch...

3/10/19
Well, this is just how things have been going lately:

Not only is my fatal disease officially rare, but the National Institutes of Health list it as an 'orphan disease', meaning it's so rare that it isn't worth anybody's time and money to research treatments for it, because they just won't make their sacred R & D costs back. #timetobuyabunchofpowerball tickets

Me: There's something a LITTLE funny about a teacher used to flunking lazy students getting heart 'failure.'

Me: I think I'll start calling mine 'acute cardiac passage.'

Me: At least ATTR has an A in it.

Nancy: Heart failure isn't usually fast.

Me: No, but it's certain.

Dave: Well, there goes the 12 hours of rapier and dagger marathon...

Jill: I appreciate your humor in the face of something this unfunny.

Me: No point in moping. I'm already taking Wellbutrin for that.

Barbara: How is your family dealing with all this?

Me: Not as well as I am, oddly.

Maria: Is transplant still an option?

Me: Going to see the big regional expert at noon today to get all of the options.

Maria: Good. It ain't over until the fat lady sings. As far as I'm concerned, the fat lady is not even clearing her throat yet.

Me: He says if they end up doing that (not imminent), at least the liver can stay.

'Not imminent.' I should go into stand-up comedy.

3/11/19
Off to the ginormous Denver Anschutz Medical Center (Disneyland for the Doomed) so the big expert on my rare condition can tell me just how screwed I am: immediately 'might as well rob a bank because you'll be dead before trial' or only 'mostly dead' and I can kick Humperdink's ass first.

He's the bad guy in 'The Princess Bride.' Miracle Max was not a fan.

Me: I should at the least score a handicapped parking sticker out of this, so it's not a TOTAL loss.

Julie: I suggest you not pay more for the fast lane.

Aleks: If you do end up robbing that bank, don't forget about your students (especially the poor ones).

Me: Suck it up, snowflake. I'm giving you a priceless education.

Me: Looks like I can kick Humperdink's ass first, but they're scheduling a fancy-shmancy pulmonary/cardiac stress test first, and maybe running a catheter into my beating heart to check its pumping pressure.

The Cardiac Wing of the Anschutz Medical Center has the swankiest waiting room of any hospital I've ever seen. In fact, it's more upscale than any hotel I've ever been in. But since everybody sitting in it has some serious life-threatening shit wrong with them, a nice waiting area is the least they could do.

But your average hotel lobby doesn't have 37 bottles of complementary hand sanitizer.

That cardiologist (Dr. Ambardekar) was awfully damned matter-of-fact about a potential heart transplant down the road. You'd have thought he was an account talking about changes to the tax law.

Eileen: Just because a surgeon is a brilliant technician doesn't mean he's a compassionate man. In fact, many of the best surgeons I knew could easily have been on the spectrum. Doesn't help when you're sitting in the chair across from him, though.

Me: I suppose that's better than having a doctor who freaks out at stuff.

Maria: I deal with cardiologists all the time. Most of them are just like that. Like mechanics scheduling a car in for a tuneup. It's hard on the patients, but it's also sort of understandable — if these people tried to invest themselves emotionally into every single heart surgery they do, they probably would have gone stark raving mad in like three weeks.

Liana: Keep in mind, too, that they deal is these issues on a daily basis, especially at Anchutz. It actually is not too far afield from auto repairs.

If I'm a car, I feel like a rusty '54 DeSoto.

If I do end up needing a heart transplant, it seems my guy is the boss of the Transplant Center. Always good to have connections.

Maria: Good. We'd rather have you with the boss of the Transplant Center than some junior McDonald's burger assembler.

If those jobs were combined, though…

"I need 2 Big Macs with extra myocardium, hold the Mayo Clinic!"

The whole time the doctor was talking about a potential heart transplant, all I could think of was the 'Live Organ Transplants' scene in Monty Python's *The Meaning of Life*. (link #1)

Me: Though he says no matter what, my liver stays. #it'sthelittlethings

It's a sobering moment when your cardiologist tells you that a heart transplant is CHEAPER than the new drug that MIGHT help your condition some.

Me: FYI, they want $450,000 a year for it.

Maria: Does it come with a mansion on a ten-acre property?

Me: And drug companies wonder why we hate them more than Nazis.

Liana: Holy crap! Wondering how much it cost to make it.

Me: I'm betting $1.95 a ton.

Russell: In the U.K., that would cost me nothing and, even a younger person in full-time work would pay less than £100 per year. A heart transplant would cost none of us anything at all. I don't know how you guys manage.

Me: Most don't. I have pretty upper-crust insurance from the school district or we'd be screwed.

Barbara: Are you and the docs contemplating a heart transplant?

Me: That's the only fix for TTR amyloidosis in the long-term. Not there yet.

Cindi: When my first husband died in 1988, we donated his organs. I'm a firm believer in organ donation. If it was your kidney, I'd volunteer to be tested to see if I could be a live donor for you.

Aww.

So I went to the big-time cardiologist yesterday with a tiny forlorn hope that he'd look at the data and say, "Hey! They blew the test. You'll be fine!" But, no. He did more blood tests while I was there and I just saw them. There are 3 biomarkers that are about 100% accurate for heart damage/heart failure. One was up 800% from mid-February, when it was already too high. Another was 6 times higher than the safe limit. The third was 70% over the safe line. Plus, the

nuclear test is practically foolproof and came back positive.

Emphasis on 'practically,' as you'll see.

And how's YOUR day going?

Erin: If they are having you run on the treadmill than that is a sorry state of healthcare. The UK and other more knowledgeable countries have moved all lung/cardiac treadmill tests to be walking tests as it actually gives more accurate results. (my mother in law was head mugwump of the cardiology dept. Trust me, it should be a walking test, anyway, no matter your age or fitness level.)

Me: It's probably a walking test. This is an internationally recognized heart program. I did have to run at the end of the basic treadmill test in September, which showed nothing.

Maria: Ugh... can't they just put you on the alignment rack or something?

There is a test that's literally called 'dipstick urinalysis.' Not joking. Checks for sugar and blood.

Me: I swear, the diagnostics may kill me before the heart failure can.

Me: I'll bet this is REALLY pissing off the overpaid CEO of my insurance company.

He probably had to buy a smaller yacht this year.

Janet: It's not doing my blood pressure any good, either.

Christina: I feel for you, Terry. My son has an auto-immune disease, and sometimes it seems like the worst part is all of the tests and doctors' appointments and the ridiculousness of the American medical system. I really, really hope they can come up with a treatment plan for you.

Me: They're putting me on stuff that dilates the vessels and increases the flow, to help with the shortness of breath and chest pains. But most heart failure meds are actually counterproductive with amyloidosis.

Andrea: Damn, Terry. You know what is saving you? Your humor. Keep up the attitude, because, y'know, none of us are getting out of here alive.

3/12/19
Health tip: DON'T visit YouTube to see what they do during a heart transplant when you're looking at maybe having to be on the receiving end someday. (link #2)

Me: There's a hospital in Texas that lets you hold your old heart after they've given you the new one. I really want a selfie with my traitorous heart. That'd make it all worthwhile… almost.

Jim: You could binge on *Grey's Anatomy* or another medical-procedure show. Not really recommending that, either, though.

Me: Having lived in hospitals lately, let me tell you how little steamy romance happens there.

Me: But on the upside, literally EVERYTHING else tests at way better than somebody my age should be, so there's that.

Jim: Reminds me of a car we had, where something crapped out deep inside the engine, requiring a decision — replace the engine, or junk the car. Since the REST of the car was in good shape, we replaced the engine, and drove it for another 100K miles.

Harriet: So, afterwards we could ask for "pics or it didn't happen"?

Me: I'm guessing the 30,000 stitches would be some sort of proof.

Scott: Well, after all the years that you've left us in stitches, I suppose this might be karmic payback?

Just walked a freaking mile with NO shortness of breath, elevated pulse, or chest pains. But in class I ran out of breath standing in one place talking to the students. There's no predicting this supposedly fatal crap I have.

As far as I can tell from the video, a heart transplant is basically a friendly autopsy.

Maria: Well...I mean...considering the OTHER autopsy, it's not such a bad option, is it?

Me: It was pretty damned gruesome. I suppose one shouldn't inquire into how the sausage is made.

The worst part was cracking the sternum. Looked like splitting a piece of cheap plywood.

Toni: I know it's scary as heck, but I know two people who went through them successfully. None who didn't make it. Still, I'd be feeling exactly what you're feeling.

3/13/19
26-hour headache and counting. Great snow day.

Russell: Caused by the drugs?

Me: No, it started before I took the first heart failure med. Probably the storm's pressure change, because it's easing up now.

Around 20 doctor visits since September and more scheduled.

Just stop counting...you'll drain your calculator batteries.

3/14/19
Up at 2 freaking a.m. Headache too bad to lie down with, a bit better upright. Over 26 hours and it still hurts. Shivering like I have a fever, but my temp is actually a degree LOW. Started with the storm, so I'm really hoping it's a reaction to the abnormal barometric pressure and not some weird cardiac crap. 5 straight days now of either head cold, cough, or this. #pardonmywhining

A second snow day, a second day with this headache. I'm getting a

lawyer and suing Fate.

Turned out I could either pay him or my transplant surgeon, but not both, so…

In case anybody's still wondering: yeah, I'm a lousy patient.

Me: The wife and my doctors/nurses will be happy to confirm this.

Janet: He's a terrible patient.

3/15/19
I'm not sure that trading very occasional chest pain for a non-stop headache is a good deal with these heart failure meds.

Kelly: Is it a side-effect of meds?

Me: Yep.

Janet: You finally got rid of the headache from the storm and the head cold. You don't need pills to make it come back and fixing the headache with Tylenol seems counter-productive.

Me: Can't take Tylenol every day. Then I WOULD need a liver transplant.

Janet: The doctor said they are to make you feel better, not worse.

Me: They're only for chest pain, which happens rarely and only with exercise. They don't fix the shortness-of-breath episodes.

Janet: I'm thinking that occasional chest pain is preferable to a constant headache. They aren't for any healing benefit from what I remember him saying.

Me: Clearly it wasn't just the storm that caused the Wednesday torture. That was my first day on the meds and the next day I didn't take the pill and it all went away.

Maria: I went through three different blood pressure meds before we found one that didn't kill me outright. The first one made me vomit, the next two brought on migraines. Definitely tell your doc — you should not be going through this.

Me: Alas, it says 'side effect: headache' right on the bottle.

Me: 11 hours and counting. Tylenol hasn't touched it.

Janet: It took over 24 hours for it to go away the last time. Clearly the pills are the problem. You can discuss this at the Monday appointment.

3/16/19
The medically induced headache only lasted 16 hours this time. Tossed the meds. Good thing they only cost $8.

Rebecca: Did you tell your doctor. Yes, I will hound you.

Me: He told me they could cause headaches and it says so on the bottle. He neglected to mention that they'd last an eternity and that the Tylenol he advocated wouldn't make a dent in them.

The medical community only prescribes Tylenol. One wonders how much in bribes it's costing the mighty Tylenol corporation.

3/18/19
Apparently, I've been living in a comfy cocoon of cardiac self-delusion. I told the cardiologist today (Dr. Carlyle) that I had hardly any symptoms and a heart transplant had to be a long way off. She begged to differ and started listing off all of the blood tests, all the echocardiogram alarms, etc. until she nearly ran out of fingers. She also said that in people as 'young' as me, heart failure can be masked and you can seem a lot healthier than you actually are. The upshot was that if the upcoming cardio/pulmonary stress test and catheter inspection come back awful, they may be sticking me on the transplant list sooner rather than later.

Me: It's just weird that I'm perfectly functional, but all of the heart experts are freaking out.

Scott: How many times have you seen an audience praise a show, when you could see every flaw and near miss, and knew just how close it came to disaster? Heck, how many times have you seen an ACTOR feel better about a show's status than it deserved? A trained expert with a little distance can see many things.

Maria: While I am not hugely fond of panicky doctors, in matters but of the heart, I'd rather have them freaking out and staying on top of everything going on with you than being super-perky and missing things.

Alaena: Well, the upside is that people in Colorado can't drive for shit and hopefully your term on the transplant list will be short lived. Just think every time someone cuts you off, they might just be interviewing for your next heart.

There's a joke you get here: Why do people come to Colorado junkyards to get turn signals? Because they've never been used.

Me: Not wishing ill to anyone, but if a 25-year-old marathoner at the Olympic Training Center in Colorado Springs happens to fall down a flight of stairs...

Greta: I shouldn't have laughed, should I?

Maria: Having dealt with a loved one's transplant situation myself, I encourage you all to just relax about this new morbid aspect to your sense of humor. It will happen. Don't feel guilty. It's not your fault that this is how the process works. You know and we, your friends, know that, had there been any other way for you to get that new heart — you would have taken it. But it is what it is. So, don't feel guilty, and laugh.

Rebecca: You have to make the reunion in 2 years.

Me: Wouldn't I technically be eligible for two different reunions, then? Mine and the donor's?

I'm old enough to remember the first heart transplant in 1967. We thought it was pure science fiction. Now I have multiple doctors acting like it's basically changing a tire. #weird

Me: Though my research tells me it's absolutely NOT like that.

*Though the hourly rate of an auto mechanic **is** about the same as a transplant surgeon's.*

John: Just make sure your doctors don't lose the lug nuts once they start, and things should be fine.

They can keep their damned hands off my lug nuts and concentrate on the heart.

Dave: Thank heaven you've kept yourself in such excellent shape. You probably nailed all of the criteria for transplant.

True. They said I was their ideal candidate: crazy-healthy everywhere but the heart. If somebody's at death's door, they're unlikely to be transplanted. Won't survive surgery or recovery.

Maria: Someday, we'll get to a point where we won't even need transplants anymore. We'll be able to just send a bunch of nanites into the body, find what's wrong and fix it on the spot.

Virginia: It is still best to do it where the surgery is performed often and by a doctor who has done a lot of them.

Me: My transplant center in Denver has done over 500 of these. Currently they do about 1 a week.

Jonathan: Elsa's cousin's a heart surgeon, based at Papworth. He once said about a valve replacement, "Oh, we could do one of those on a kitchen table..."

Then an appendectomy could be done on what, a tea trolley?

I can think of better ways to get out of major SAT proctoring duty than this. But I was running out of breath just trying to tell our assistant principal why I should only be an alternate.

Andrew: Play your cards right and I hear it's about $50K a pop to take the test for them.

The kids at this top-ranked school would sneer at the thought of me taking their test, because they'd flunk the math portion by about 2,000 points.

3/19/19
Just to show you how far medicine has come since 1967, this country does 10 heart transplants a DAY now and nobody even mentions it.

And that's not even counting the extra-terrestrial scientific experiments at Area 51. #thetruthisoutthere

3/20/19
Well, normally birthdays are no big deal to me, but thanks to recent developments, suddenly I'm a lot more focused on them than I used to be.

Me: Old I am, and scarred, like Jerusalem's hills.

What? Doesn't every heart transplant memoir reference 'Moby Dick'?

It was very sweet of my students to get me a musical birthday card, but they didn't think through the awkwardness of it being one where you had to blow on the pop-up candle to activate it, since shortness of breath is one of my heart failure symptoms.

"And I'll huff, and I'll puff, and I'll…yeah, that's about it. Huff and puff."

That's me, Hufflepuff all the way.

3/21/19
Well, it's official. I've been ordered by the wife to live long enough to take her to *Harry Potter* and *Star Wars* at Disney World. #finallyarealreasontolive

Rebecca: You have to go. Just don't go in the summer.

Alaena: #lifegoals

Janet: Smith We can't go till *Star Wars Land* is finished in Orlando, which is in the fall of this year at the earliest. Universal has a new Hagrid ride that looks terrific, too. So Terry has to stay healthy until fall of 2020 at the very least.

We can't go till the geriatric basset hound shuffles off this mortal coil. The dog boarding would cost more than the trip.

Jim: Y'know, Terry, that Janet is just gonna keep coming up with this kind of thing. She's gonna have you live forever.

Janet: Yup, that's the plan.

I'll be on life-support with the family surrounding me for 'his brave last day' and she'll run in hollering, "They just opened 'Doctor Who World' in Hong Kong!"

Julie: I have a friend who drives the train in Animal Kingdom. If Terry behaves, I'll make arrangements so he can blow the train whistle. This post is meant to be read without euphemisms.

If I behave? That seems like an awfully high bar. Cut a guy some slack.

Larraine: When you guys do come to Orlando, be sure to let me know. We can meet up and I'll be your official tour guide. Moved here 12 years ago and we've done it all. Also because Travis is autistic, we get handicapped passes at the parks (quick ride lines).

Janet: That's very cool. Terry is also autistic and has a difficult time with long lines, overstimulation, and unexpected glitches. Traveling in general is something he loves, but he doesn't understand that it makes me so stressed that I don't enjoy the vacation time. I never know when the next meltdown will happen. The blood pressure meds can only do so much. At least at Disney parks, it's clean and orderly and they take care of a lot of the details. Plus, he can go to the room and take a nap if it gets to be too much and I can still play.

Larraine: Terry and Travis would get along great. Travis is 18 now and a real treasure of info on all the parks. He watches YouTube non-stop, gathering info on different parks history, secrets, what's to come, etc. It's his thing.

Janet: I can't think of a better thing to research than Disney parks. Terry's so into his medical problems and researching them that it's making me crazy. I can handle blood and physical problems, but invisible diseases make me queasy. We would love to say hello sometime. Depends on how the heart problems turn out.

3/23/19
Dr. Carlyle made me go back on the vasodilation meds from hell that gave me a 26-hour headache. At least she's letting me cut them in half and only take them every other day to start. It's a dull ache so far, much better than before. Hopefully, the duration will be less, too.

Michael: Soooo... Super Viagra?

Me: Um...not so much.

Though that would've made it easier for me to bear, Janet likely would've fled in terror at the prospect. #stayawayfrommewiththatthing

3/25/19
Managed to walk 2.25 miles today without chest pain or shortness of breath, but the pulse rate on the second mile, same pace, DOUBLED for no obvious reason to 151. That's 95% of maximum while walking an 18-minute mile. So the treadmill stress test at the hospital on Wednesday looks like it'll be...interesting.

Me: FYI, I **ran** BolderBoulder with a lower pulse rate.

3/26/19
10 slow miles on the bike, first ride since February 2. No health issues. At least I don't have to sell this $4000+ worth of stuff yet. Top-shelf bicycle components are in the same price range as medical technology.

3/27/19
The hospital DNA test came back negative for familial (mutant)

TTR amyloidosis, so I have what's called the wild form. Means I don't have to freak out the relatives by telling them they have to get tested.

Fun as it would've been to call them up in faux-panic screaming, "You're all doomed! Doomed!"

And for those who might be disappointed that I'm not officially a mutant...there's still plenty of wiggle room on that.

Harriet: You wild child, you!

Jeanne: So, if it's not genetic, does that mean you caught it somehow?

Me: It's genetic, just not inherited. Simple bad luck. Not contagious.

Maria: I was just going to say — I feel lonely being the only mutant among the people I know. Get a move on, will ya?

Make sure to tell me where and when they have the membership meetings.

Mark: I was about to say...haven't you been a mutant for a long time now?

Me: You're not wrong.

Fasting for 4 hours to prep for my VO/2 stress treadmill test at 1p.m., aka 'The World's Most Expensive Walk to Nowhere.'

'__Fasting__' for a slow walk. Doesn't get better than that for an English teacher.

Back from the treadmill stress test at Cardiology Central. They seemed impressed at how long and hard I managed to walk on the thing. They put it up at a fast pace up a 12% gradient. As I was congratulating myself on that, the nurse said, "You'd be surprised how many marathon runners I get in here for heart transplants."

Me: 10 miles on the bike yesterday, no problem. Treadmill test, no problem.

Just walking in the door of the hospital to take the test: chest pains. WTF?

Julie: You are playing by rules you've never encountered before.

Me: Clearly. The test was so easy, at this point I'm expecting the actual result to be horrific.

CS: There's a story of a Chinese doctor who is asked how to prolong life. He answers: 'The heart is a pump. Like any pump, it's only good for so many compressions. You run, your heart beats faster, making more compressions. You want to live longer? Take a nap.'

Dee: Giant tortoises live a long time.

Mandy: So there's something to be said for the sedentary life of a writer.

Except the heavy drinking and paralyzing self-doubt undermine it.

3/28/19
Well, they posted the results of the fancy dancy stress test already. Still looking up what all of the jargon means, but those two 'severely abnormals' are pretty clear.

Me: And apparently those are precisely the ones you DON'T want to be abnormal.

Me: But some of the others are perfect. Weird.

Fate was just having its little joke.

3/30/19
They're planning on running a catheter into my beating heart, just to see if maybe there are a few gnomes living there, I guess. #gnomeremovalclinicaltrial

Liana: Ask if you can watch the monitor with them.

I did, later, during biopsies. Seeing the probe snake into the heart, and also feeling it skip a beat as it went through the valve, was...thrilling.

Mark: Won't feel a thing, and the sensation of peeing yourself is highly over-rated.

Kelly: They already diagnosed you, so why all these tests?

Rebecca: The info that the heart cath will give is different than all the other tests. It is usually done after all the other tests. I would have been surprised if they didn't do one.

Iris: Gremlins?

To access the photos/videos/links:
www.terrykroenungink.com/246-2/

3) SO, A 167 RESTING PULSE IS TOO HIGH, HUH?

MARCH 30-APRIL 7, 2019

This part really jacks-up the drama, if you like emergency defibrillation, 7-hour cardiac ablations, shocking announcements from doctors, and heroic cardiac intervention.

Not to mention bison meatloaf, Shakespearean strippers, and being ogled by teams of nurses while peeing into a bottle.

By the end of March I'd been expensively tested in ways unimaginable a few weeks before. The results were mixed. A lot of them were worrisome, if you were an experienced cardiologist and knew the signs. But some, like my treadmill stress test, seemed okay. Plus, I was managing to exercise at a level that hardly indicated imminent mortality. 4 days before being rushed into a hospital bed again, I rode 10 miles on the bike in a perfectly normal pace, without any heart symptoms.

And then I ended up with an electrical scorch mark on my chest (yes, they really do holler, "Clear!" before they zap you, though "♫ Greased lightning!" would be cooler).

I spent this entire section in the Cardiac Intensive Care Unit of the Anschutz Medical Center, run by the University of Colorado Medical School. That means my room was frequently full of newly minted doctors who looked like they arrived at the hospital via skateboard.

The place is named after Philip Anschutz, the gazillionaire who gave them some of his gazillions to build the thing. His right-wing politics make me itch (that's okay, the Prednisone helped with it), but I can't say that he didn't get great results with his investment. I was awash in cardiac competence (yes, even the skateboard kids). It's a huge campus, with multiple buildings called Pavilions so they can pretend it's a happy theme park: Inpatient, Outpatient, Cancer, Eye, etc. And they're adding more. Not sure what the new ones will be for. 'Medical Bill-Induced Strokes', maybe. With all of the cash spent, precious little of it went for parking, of course. You could perish of your tragic condition driving around the lot in the vain hope that somebody would pull out. They should have old-school carhop/residents on roller skates servicing the lots with trays of meds and stethoscopes.

3/30/19
Off to the ER again. Pulse just jumped up to 167, while sitting on the couch doing nothing, chest pains not going away.

Shit.

Dave: Argh. I'll have my fingers, toes, eyes, testicles, and butt heels crossed that you get the best care and are released quickly.

3/31/19
Ventricular tachycardia that wouldn't stop. IV meds in the ER barely touched it.

So I got my first full-blown defibrillation. 200 glorious joules of electricity. Another warm spring break memory.

That was one of the thousand unnatural shocks that flesh is heir to.

For those who didn't look it up: yes, it can kill you dead if untreated.

*The med biz calls it v tach. Sustained heartbeat over 120 when not exercising. It's sustained if it lasts more than 30 seconds. **Mine lasted over 2 hours.** That can make it go into ventricular fibrillation (the heartbeat goes spastic and then it all stops; survival rate of only 45%, even in a hospital. The ER tried 2 separate infusions of anti-arrhythmic meds to stop it. Nada. Thus the shock.*

Me: They sedated me first, thank Odin. I have no memory of it.

Just a splendid burnt spot. The Mark of Lidocaine.

Me: FYI, Fentanyl is dangerously good shit. It's as scary as the news reports say.

Tim: I've been there. VT more times than I can count. Fortunately, I had an ICD after the first time. I was only shocked a few times. The other times I was paced out of them.

Me: Looks like I'll be leaving here with an ICD, the way everybody's talking.

Tim: That's a good thing. Hopefully, it will be able to pace you out of any VT. Getting shocked is no fun.

Me: So I hear.

After stabilizing my heart by 'shocking the hell out of it' (the doctor's words), they threw me in an ambulance and zipped me to Denver. So now I'm in the Cardiac ICU at Anschutz Medical Center. And how is YOUR weekend going?

Kelly: What's going on?!

Me: Just a near-death heart episode last night. My rare disease is showing off.

"Oh, you thought that walking pulse in the 150's was something? Watch this."

The full glorious spectacle of moi post-heart shock in the Longmont ER, flying high on Fentanyl. (photo 18)

Hannah: Why does it say you're LONG?

That either means Long's Peak Hospital or it's a size-long BP cuff. There's a third possibility, but modesty doesn't permit me...

Theresa: Keep your head high and your morphine or Fentanyl higher.

There are signs in all of the UC Health facilities statewide that claim that you can get addicted to opioids in as little as 5 days. They gave them to me for 17.

They may be giving me a new pacemaker tomorrow, one with a built-in defibrillator to shock the crap out of me if things go sideways again.

Tim: I had one for 8 years. They took it out when I got the transplant.

Took my old one out, too. I hope it's an alien tech prop on some movie set now.

Looks like this won't be a one-night hospital stay like last month. Cardiac catheterization tomorrow and then probably the upscaled pacemaker. The food had better be good here.

It was, oddly enough.

My nurse is French, with a full-blown 'ain't been here that long' accent. The first cardiologist was a resident who looked like she was still in high school and was homecoming queen.

Hannah: Enjoy the female company, if anything. XX

Me: Hospitals are SO not like *Grey's Anatomy*. America needs to know this.

Maria: They could at least wear French maid outfits. Just to cheer you up a bit.

Me: Another bunch of cardio hotties just came through. I swear some pathetic guy is approving med school applications here for dubious reasons. They all know their shit, though.

I don't care if they look like Medusa, so long as they know their way around a heart, which they did.

Christine: You are a rare oddity that the kiddies may only get to see once or twice in a career, thus the parade. Docs do love their anomalies. When my sister was diagnosed with CLL, the oncologist excitedly asked if she could submit a paper about familial blood cancers (my dad died of a different variant of leukemia) right on the heels of the diagnosis.

Beth: Time to get started on this as a next book.

I hear and I obey. So let it be 'written', so let it be done.

They're starting heart transplant paperwork.

Yeah, that just happened.

Tim: That's good. They can list you at level six until you actually need a new heart. Or is their intention to get you listed and keep you there until they find a you a heart?

Me: Sounded like she was saying stay on the list until I qualify, building up seniority on the list in the meantime.

Tim: That's the path I took. Originally listed as level six back in June 2018. On December 20th I was moved up to level two. Six days later I had the transplant surgery.

Theresa: The good news is that you are not the first. You aren't even the 1000th. They are doing at least 1 a day now.

Me: This hospital has done over 500.

Veronica: Don't have the words, dude! Keeping you in my thoughts, and hey, if I see any specific jerks who might make for ideal candidates...(I am kidding, of course, in case any authority types are reading).

*I'll be lucky if **anybody** is reading this, much less authority types.*

Me: You seem young and healthy. Feel free to help a brother out.

Curtis: When obtaining a new heart make sure you get one that's still under warranty and has had the full 20-point inspection.

Me: So...not yours, then.

Curtis: Dude, everyone knows I'm heartless.

Karen: You have got this. The shock will wear off and you will begin to imagine the life you will have after you get the new heart. If you have questions let me know. I am 4-year post-transplant.

Toni: I hate that you're going through this, Terry, but two acquaintances went through this with great success. I echo everyone else's sentiments. Thoughts and prayers all around you!

Andrea: Meanwhile the Universal Heart keeps on beating...

This hospital has bison meatloaf. #mostcoloradothingever

Me: They're trying to buffalo me into ordering it.

Maria: I think you should. You know how New Zealand cannibal tribes believed that eating your enemy imbued you with all of his virtues — strength, courage, sexual prowess, etc.? Based on that, just think of the potential advantages of eating some bison! Just saying...

If I acquire the sexual prowess of a bison, Janet is outta here.

Because that would be a downgrade for me.

Jim: Well, I think that to get the most benefit, you need the eat the HEART of the enemy... or perhaps, just get a bison heart for your transplant.

Max: Nice. How is it?

Me: Didn't order it. Maybe tonight. Just for the conversation value.

Me: (later) Almost a steak texture, not like traditional meatloaf.

So...Troponin is a thing they blood-test for that indicates heart damage. It's supposed to read as almost non-existent, a reading of less than .04.

Mine is 4.56.

Me: This just gets better and better.

Me: Last month it was .12. March 11 it was .96.

Matthew: Get thee to an emergency room, if you're not already in a hospital.

Me: I'm in a Cardiac ICU as we speak.

Matthew: Now that I've read more of your posts, I can tell that you have been having your health seen to.

Me: I'm so seen to that it's starting to get absurd.

Maria: Well, it's official. You are a mutant.

I'm one of the ex-men. I have an explanted heart (that's what removing the old one is called, medically).

Beth: Eat the bison!!

Other than an in-bed echocardiogram, it looks like all I'm doing is sitting here watching my IV drip all day.

The fun never stops. #world'smostexpensivehotelroom

Shannon: Netflix was made for this.

Me: No chill, though.

Shannon: No — you oughta wait for that.

They let me get out of bed and sit in a chair, but there's literally an alarm under my ass to keep me from moving unless they help. #ourlawyersmadeusdoit

"All right, Kroenung, we've got you surrounded! Surrender quietly. Come out with your bedpans up."

Not the fastest kitchen in this hospital. Ordered breakfast over an hour ago. It's lunch time now.

Maria: Brunch. Let's call it brunch.

Samantha: I've stayed at Anshutz over twenty times since I was a kid. And I can tell you that if you even think about starting to get hungry, order then.

I quickly learned that the average wait time was 45-60 minutes. Apparently when you order chicken, they drive to a farm, select the proper egg, wait for it to reach adulthood, and then wring its neck to order.

No happy meds, just diuretics, so I need to find the little 'piddle here' bottle. (photo 19)

You may think caffeine sends you to the bathroom more often, but industrial-grade IV diuretics should be classed as military weapons.

These guidelines were created in the 1980s by Dr. Barbara Phillips, Professor of Pulmonary, Critical Care, and Sleep Medicine at the University of Kentucky College of Medicine. They are still applicable today. (photo 20)

Only Day 1 of this extended hospitalization and I'm already reduced to watching competitive Canadian axe throwing on ESPN.

Me: Yes, it's a thing. They're unbelievably accurate.

Remind me to never piss off a Canadian.

Scott: For one of Heather's infusions, we found ourselves watching the national lumberjack championships.

Did the winner sing: ♫ *"I'm a lumberjack and I'm okay,*

"I sleep all night and infuse all day…"?

Eileen: You sure you should be watching that with a dicey heart? I mean, the excitement and all.

Liana: You might want to switch to curling.

Me: If only. I actually belong to a curling league.

Much less cutting-off of toes…most of the time.

Beth: Who's winning?!

Me: Some old guy in a kilt.

Beth: Oh, good…at least he's stylish.

Jim: Ask the staff to check the channels for you. Pretty sure there's a channel dedicated to growing grass (just regular, not the Colorado kind), and perhaps, if you're very lucky, you can get the paint-drying channel.

Me: They have two channels that are just elevator music over nature videos.

Giselle: Have you access to a Kindle? That might be worth getting brought to the hospital.

Me: I'm doing all of this on the iPad the school gave me. I put a Kindle app on it.

And by 'gave" I actually mean 'forced to accept on pain of termination.'

Sheila: Watch a whole night of the Gardening Channel when I was in the hospital. You'd think with something that boring, I would have slept.

Boring? Gardening? Have you seen the implements of death they use?

Theresa: Thank you for bringing us on your journey. Its educational and brings awareness but also, it's funny and emotional and weird.

4/1/19
My blood oxygen/pulse monitor. I tried to fix my heart like ET's finger, but it didn't work. (photo 21)

"Ouuuuch…"

Rebecca: You must be getting good drugs.

Me: Just saline and Lidocaine drips, alas.

"'Tis is extempore, from my mother wit." – 'The Taming of the Shrew'

"A wit by folly vanquished. – 'Two Gentlemen of Verona'

So, of course, on the first night in a hospital ever where I was getting sustained sleep, they come in at 4 freaking a.m. to jab me with a needle…twice.

Francine: I've never had any rest in any of my hospital "visits." {{{hugs}}}

In any other circumstance this would be felonious assault. Here I pay them for the privilege.

They might have mentioned yesterday that this heart catheter thing requires me getting no food or even water. Looks like I get to go a full 24 @#$!! hours without eating or drinking.

A paltry wait. My heart transplant foodless zone was 50 hours.

Scott: I know you have a dry wit, but good grief.

Maria: But…the bison burger…

Just had an echocardiogram. I know this means nothing to all but a

couple of people here, but my left ventricular ejection fraction is half what it was only 7 weeks ago and WAY below normal. 2 years ago it was 65%, high normal, and now it's 24%. "Function severely reduced," the report says. FYI, 30% is the 'Danger! Danger, Will Robinson!' point.

No wonder the left ventricle blew out Saturday night.

Me: FYI, that's a measure of how well your heart pumps blood out to your body. That's what the left ventricle does. Too low and your whole system crashes. This IS too low.

Me: The uber-senior doctor (Dr. Wolfel) I just talked to said some of that might be 'just' due to the near-fatal tachycardia event, but only the catheterization will say for sure.

Bonnie: I was a critical care nurse for 38 years. I get it, and my thoughts and prayers are with you.

Rebecca: Please help me yell at him when he goes off of his prescribed meds.

Me: Sounds like someone may have warned them.

Tim: My EF was 18% prior to the transplant. The new and improved model is at 65%.

Well, when you get over 60 you do have trouble with your ejections.

I was kind of hoping that the roomful of doctors who were just here would say "April Fool" and send me home with 2 aspirin and a clean bill of health, but no such luck.

"Transplant it is, bucko." At least the main guy I talk to (Dr. Wolfel), older than me and apparently a high muckety-muck here, is a marathon runner and sympathizes with how much this all pisses me off. He talks about doing a heart transplant like it's easier than putting up a bouncy castle.

Julie: I don't know. Some of those bouncy castles are pretty complex.

Me: Looks like I'm here all week regardless of what heart procedures they do. The pre-transplant tests are apparently epic and will take until Thursday.

Alaena: Easier to get them out of way and done in one trip.

Tim: I agree. I did mine as an outpatient and it took a month to get them all in.

Me: If I hadn't just been running 10K's and biking 100 miles at a shot, I wouldn't be so annoyed.

Me: It's a rough way to have ice-breaker conversation at parties.

(Opening shirt) "You might want to finish eating that, ma'am."

Dai: Well, it's not **brain** surgery.

Maria: As long as he doesn't try to do the transplant WHILE on the bouncy castle, we should be okay.

Maria: Terry mentioned *Grey's Anatomy* in an earlier post (or two). In that show, they've done surgery during hurricanes, floods, in sink holes, in active-shooter situations, and all kinds of other stuff. Pretty sure they didn't do bouncy castle, though. Unless you wanna count earthquake. I think they did earthquake.

Maria: If I absolutely had to choose, I'd rather have *House M.D.*

Not a great example for fixing the current opioid epidemic, though.

Alaena: Mom and I were talking about *House M.D.* today. Pretty sure they did your disease at least a few times.

Already signed the first transplant paperwork, so we're off to the races.

Apparently, I have the good blood type for this, so that's something.

Christina: My dad had a heart transplant in 1989 and he's still going strong at 86 years old. You can do this.

Well, the heart transplant games have begun. I just had TWENTY (not hyperbole) vials of blood drawn at once.

Me: All off of a single stick to the vessel, thankfully. This nurse is a trained professional.

Me: The stool sample will be a fun experience.

*Good thing they didn't want 20 of **those**.*

Christine: Okay, I give up. What does analyzing your own personal Poop Monster have to do with a heart transplant? Oh, wait, I remember.

'Anal'yzing. (snicker)

Yes, I'm an actual adult role model for America's youth.

Julia: You must have forgotten the garlic to keep the vampires away.

Kate: Whoa! Hey, maybe they want less blood in their way?

Cindi: I hope you're taking notes so you can write a book about all this. As horrific as this situation is, your Facebook posts and attitude are quite entertaining.

Tim: I remember that. A number of them are for infectious disease. They want to try and ensure that you are immunized against certain diseases since your immune system will be suppressed after the transplant. Hopefully, the ablation will be successful and you end up not needing a transplant.

Me: There's no way out of the transplant. They have no cure for what I have, they've made that very clear more than once today. All that's up in the air is how many months or years they can wait.

Months…how innocent I was back then.

Tim: Got it. Hopefully you get listed quickly. Do you think they will want you to stay in the hospital until a match is found?

Me: I don't think they're under that much of a time crunch. They just want me on the list so my clock can start ticking.
"Not much of a time crunch." (turns purple laughing)

Getting an ablation tomorrow (going in with a catheter to basically cauterize the spot that tried to kill me Saturday). Maybe ALL of tomorrow. They say it could take as long as 7 hours. A Catheter Lab looks like this. (photo 22)

And that's precisely how long they poked around in there. Must get paid by the hour.

Me: At least this one has a scheduled start time and I know to eat and drink a ton before the midnight cutoff.

Tim: I had 3 ablations. I was under for 16 hours for the last one. Fingers crossed that the ablation is successful.

Karen: My ablation was at Brigham & Women's Hospital in Boston, on the day of the Boston Marathon bombing. Hubby was walking downtown and made it just inside the hospital entrance before the SWAT team locked everything down and brought one of the bombers to the hospital. Good times.

There were days that I felt my hospital room was a crime scene.

20 blood draws, an abdominal ultrasound, and an information session about an LVAD (left ventricular assist device) in the past 90 minutes. Waiting for the lower extremity inspector to show. They aren't messing around with this pre-transplant stuff.

Maria: Basically, you are going to feel like a car needing the engine replaced.

Christine: LVADs are actually pretty cool things, especially if they keep your ticker tocking along until a new one is found.

I wanted no part of an LVAD unless there was no choice. They crack you open and basically carve out the inside of your heart and install a pump, with an exterior motor and about 10 lbs. of batteries that you wear on a vest 24/7. Lots of infections and other problems, too. It's like an uncool, unweaponed Iron Man.

The big transplant conference is happening now in Orlando, Florida ("Your destination experience for invasive orthotopic allografts"). I kid you not, one of the panels is called "Making Co-morbidities Great Again." #thosewhackytransplanters

One imagines the wild after-hours parties where they offer CPR to strippers.

Maria: You are writing all this down as book ideas, yes?

Me: More or less.

Day 3. The rollicking adventure continues.

Jim: You're in dubiously good company. Mick Jagger had to put a tour on hold to get heart surgery.

Me and Mick are tight like that.

Me: I can't get no satisfaction here, either.

Curtis: You have my sympathy, you devil.

Not used to shaving around a gaping hole in my jugular vein.

Jim: Well — I know this guy on Fleet Street who could shave you. He's used to dealing with jugulars.

♫ *"My friends, my faithful friends…"*

'Sweeney Todd, the Demon Barber of Fleet Street', for those not well-versed in 19ᵗʰ century Grand Guignol.

4/2/19
It's that nifty 2:20 a.m. hospital update you've all been waiting for.

Awake at 1:50 to piddle into a bottle so they can measure my output, because that's how things roll here. But the ventricular tachycardia alarm went off for 10 whole seconds and the nurse freaked, so I got thrown back into bed while she paged (apparently that's still a thing) my heart failure team to get permission for me to pee. Then while I was up anyway, why not jab me with a needle, because the previous 20 vials of blood weren't enough. I'm amazed there's any left. I should like a giant pasty old prune by now.

I should've looked like the victims of the salt vampire in 'Star Trek.'

Mandy: Would you please stop scaring the nurses! They'll do more than vampirise you if you're not careful...((healing hugs))

Literally true, dear.

Maria: What would have happened if they didn't give you permission to pee?

Me: They're not the boss of me. #rebelwithoutapot

61 years old and people stand around me encouraging me to excrete like I'm a toddler. #who'sagoodboy?

Janet: You and Abby are getting the same treatment.

Abby's our 10-year-old basset hound. She won't go if it's wet outside.

Me: I ain't goin' out to pee in the rain, either, lady.

Peter: I am so glad you have kept up your sense of humour. Believe me it helps!

Karen: Let me tell you a story. After my transplant I had a few complications, led to a week-long coma that set me back in the motor skills department. I could not talk at first and I could not move my hands, arms, legs, feet. So the goal was to move something. Anything. Mayo is a great hospital, but I'd had just about enough. Don't they think I would have moved if I could? FFS. So, my new doctor (all of a week with his MD), I like to call him Rico Suave, comes in with about 12 interns and a couple of his SR doctors. He is pushing, and threatening, and cajoling and I reached my breaking point. Still unable to talk, I did what he wanted. I MOVED ONE FINGER. Guess which finger? The entire pack of doctors almost peed themselves and my husband just groaned. LOL

It's amazing how quickly you can get used to piddling into a bottle next to your bed, in front of a giant window with a spectacular view of the Rocky Mountains, while having a casual conversation with ladies you've never met, who have to observe the whole thing in case you pass out.

No performance anxiety here. "Let me share this magnificence with the world!"

The new night nurse looks like one of my high school students. So does the other night nurse and several of my cardiologists. They must be sending them to college when they're 14.

Me: Or maybe I'm just so old now that practically everybody looks like an infant.

Me: New day nurse, same deal.

'I'll lay 14 of my teeth…she is not 14." – 'Romeo and Juliet'

'Fecal occult blood' is a real thing.

Me: I'm negative for that, BTW. That's a good thing, because otherwise I'd have to sacrifice a virgin to my colon.

Maria: A virgin what? Human, goat, monkey, a dozen fruit flies?

Liana: Maybe a bottle of virgin olive oil. That's the only virgin I've seen or heard about recently.

Fiona: In what way is it occult? Can one use it for demon summoning????

Me: *Bell, Book, and Colon.*

Me: *Harry Potter and the Sorcerer's Stool.*

Tom Sawyer's Aunt Polyp. Sailing across the Pacific to French Polypnesia. The Greeks and Spartans fighting the Polypennisian War.

Andrea: Good name for a heavy metal band.

Didn't see that coming from an opera singer. I'd pay top dollar to see you sing with Ozzy.

Stephanie: I am so sorry you're sick, but your feed is one of the most entertaining things on FB right now!

Dai: Here in Scotland we over 60's get to send stool samples to Dundee every two years to test for just that.

Who did poor Dundee piss off???

Guess who has a lovely scorch mark on his chest from being defibrillated Saturday night?

This guy, that's who. Don't be jealous. Envy is an ugly thing.

Veronica: Too late. My eyes radiate green.

Xiaoyi: Photos? I know I ask for odd things.

Rebecca: Beats the alternative.

Me: Well, yeah.

Alaena: Pics or it didn't happen.

Oh, it happened, all right. Your mom was on the other side of the curtain, freaking out, when they hollered, "Clear!"

Dean: Stop lying. That's where they removed the xenomorph from you, isn't it?

Xenomorphs remove themselves.

Garalt: If this is an elaborate wind-up, I know a good lawyer you could hire.

Sorry, all my money is going for sets, costumes, and actors playing doctors.

Maria: Now you have a legitimate excuse to say, "You should see the other guy."

Karen: I have no scars from that. Mine was an implant and before my transplant the freaking thing went off about 40+ times...in my chest. Gack!

Off for a heart ablation. See you all on the other side.

Julie: You know I get lost easily.

Just follow the hospital admin people chasing me with release forms to sign.

Sarah: May they aim like a Jedi, not a Storm Trooper.

"Aren't you a little short to be a cardiologist?"

Maria: Ok, it's been 8 hours. Any word?

Theresa: Terry, I hope you're just really, really high right now and that nothing has happened.

Me: Not high at all. That all wore off ages ago. Just an awful hangover from the anesthesia. Feels worse than the heart issue that put me here.

7 hours on the operating table. Took them a long time to find the bad spot causing the tachycardia and burn it out with a probe. Then they tried to force me into tachycardia at that same place to be sure they

got it. 4 hours after that, forced to lie flat on my back, unmoving, while they kept tabs on the ginormous holes they punched in my groin to run the catheters through. Have a headache and semi-nausea like the world's worst hangover. Oh...a foot-long catheter up into your tender old bladder isn't as much fun as it sounds. #thisdayprettymucksucked

And, of course, it all turned out to be completely unnecessary, as they threw the heart away five days later.

Leah: So glad to see your snarky words on here.

Harriet: Being here to bitch about it is a good sign.

Liana: Be glad they made you lie flat. You DIDN'T want to sit up after that, trust me.

Jim: Me: when do you take the catheter out? Doc: Oh, I don't. Here's instructions on how you can do it yourself at home. Me: Dafu...?

Had a nurse do it. Burned like the fires of Hades.

Mark: Foot long?! Boaster!

Hey, tape measures don't lie…

Maria: They don't just owe you some bison stew. They owe you a seven-course dinner with dancing girls.

I don't think I could digest more than 3 dancing girls.

Julie: Glad to find my snark update this morning.

Tim: Hopefully the ablation is successful. I actually forgot about the whole groin thing. I think I blocked it out.

The undignified manscaping on the table was a special treat.

After 7 hours of being probed inside the heart, that's actually the only

place where I'm not miserable. I mean, you'd think you'd feel SOMETHING there.

Samantha: Haven't felt anything in that region for years!

Shannon: Does this mean you are spiritually heartless?

In hindsight, it's probably a really good thing I didn't feel anything there. Not that it mattered much, since that was Tuesday and they trash-canned it on Sunday.

4/3/19
I TOLD you I was sick! (photo 23)

David: Good grief, man! Even Darth Vader doesn't have that much equipment in his cocoon.

The post-transplant machines made this paltry equipment look like a 90's cellphone.

Me: This is nothing. The cardiac ablation lab looks like NASA Command Central.

And the transplant OR looks like the inside of a Bond villain's hollow volcano.

Julie: Do you have the machine that goes ping?

Me: Every damned thing here pings, chirps, or buzzes.

Ironically, in Chinese, 'ping' means 'sound of crashing.'

Julie: Tell them it would increase your sense of well-being if they were all tuned to the same key.

Jacqueline: OMG SOMEONE GOT THERE FIRST.

Ana: Is that your new android heart?

John: His iOS iHeart won't be ready until next week. It'll be much more streamlined, and actually fit in his chest.

But the charger comes separately and the device isn't as good as a Galaxy S10.

Veronica: We assumed you meant in the head.

Me: If they try to transplant that, too, I'll fight them tooth and claw.

Unless they have a better-looking one in stock. With hair. Then I'd have to think about it.

Christina: I like your yellow socks.

Rebecca: Do not ever put a bare foot on a hospital floor. I am glad to see the foot covered.

I'm not crazy. I know what's on a hospital floor. Rather lick a toilet seat.

Garalt: Are you powering all that equipment?

With my vast intellect, yes.

Kate: Wow, that's a weird art installation you got in that overpriced hotel room.

When they watch me pee, its performance art.

Hannah: Oh, Terry! You are magnificent! What special heart will suit your personality, I wonder?

Me: Smart-ass Olympic marathon runner would-be good.

Looks like I'm going on the transplant list after the meeting tomorrow, unless something changes. Level 4, most likely. Priority is 1 & 2.

Pete: That's gotta be a positive development, albeit daunting, if not terrifying. I think this is what they mean by the night being darkest before the dawn.

You can literally transplant an entire heart in the time it took them to cauterize a couple of millimeters of tissue in mine yesterday.

Tim: True.

Eileen: Transplanting is easier. You don't have to find that one, teeny-tiny, weensy-bitty piece of pacemaking tissue out of every other cell of pacemaking tissue to target.

Russell: God, you're always complaining...

Hey, I'm the customer here. It's my natural right.

And you can get to the moon with less tech than in a cardiac ablation lab.

Bill: Actually, the first microprocessor was not invented when we landed on the moon. The astronauts used a slide-rule, paper and space-pens to calculate. The computers back then were very crude by today's standards. I have several magnitudes more power in my smartwatch than they had at NASA.

Go ahead, kids, Google 'slide rule.' We'll wait. (pause) Wild, huh?

Liana: The "computers" were women.

This is true. Unappreciated women.

Russell: 32k to the moon and back.

Pete: There was a delay in the launch of Apollo 9 when they lost the key to wind it up with.

Nanci: When I had my ablation ten years ago, I had to be awake to give feedback. It was like being a patient on *House*.

Me: That was sort of the original plan, but then the thing got too long and involved, so they just put me all the way out.

Time to snooze in this epically overpriced (this week may run over $150,000) and over staffed (8 doctors in here at a time; one has 43 years of medical experience) hotel room. Tomorrow I get a fancy new pacemaker with the new bonus feature of shocking the crap out of my heart if goes into arrhythmia. They say I should go home Friday.

And 8 weeks of not being allowed to lift my left arm. Good thing I don't use it to write snarky Facebook posts.

Tim: I've been there. You'll find that it's nice having an ICD, unless it's shocking you too often.

They cancelled that. And they aren't letting me leave, either. The Transplant Committee just met, and they all agree that I have to get listed right freaking now and wait in this bed until it's go time, no matter how long it takes.

Me: That was a hell of a way to wake up.

Rebecca: Please keep up with the snark. I get worried if you go too long without snarking.

Me: The snark is strong with this one.

'Snark' comes from Lewis Carroll, of course. It's a combination of snake and shark. It comes from his nonsense poem "The Hunting of the Snark", which is appropriately subtitled "An agony in eight fits." That perfectly describes my hospital experience.

Christine: You do know all those doctors are stopping by because you are so big a medical anomaly that this may be their only chance to see a case. Charge each a small fee and you might even be able to buy your insurance company.

I need to charge them more than a small fee just to break even. Most of them bill over $400 just for crossing my threshold.

4/4/19
(Janet) Terry's got one more procedure left to go and if it goes as planned, he can leave the hospital tomorrow. He needs a pacemaker

upgrade. Hopefully, sometime this morning.

Or...not.

Me: It's cancelled, dear. You need to get here ASAP.

Janet: I know. I just talked to the nurse practitioner. We'll be there as soon as Alaena gets back from walking the dogs. She said that you are off food restrictions. Anything you want us to get you on the way?

Well, a barely-used heart would be nice, now that you mention it.

Me: Nail clippers.

Weirdly, my nurses weren't allowed to cut my toenails. Something about liability if they accidentally cut me. Remember, this is a place that punctures you daily to take blood, and guts you like a fish to yank out your heart, with only one signature on a form.

Well, this day went sideways in a hurry.

Long story short: no ICD implantation at all. They strolled in at 8 a.m. and announced that not only am I not leaving tomorrow, I'm not leaving at all. The Transplant Committee is jumping me up the list and keeping me here. They think I'm way closer to being dead than I feel. Dr. Ambardekar came back from his transplant conference in Florida and overruled everybody. Which is weird, because they took me off all the IV's and monitors, except a wireless heart monitor, and are letting me stroll around the hospital. No idea how long before this happens. Days, weeks, months. Absolutely best case: back teaching in the fall. Worst case: one whack-a-doodle memorial service (I want strippers and Shakespeare scenes).

Maria: Let's put it this way - you ARE leaving there at some point. On your own two feet. Because those Shakespearean strippers don't come cheap — think of all the underskirts and corsets they have to go through.

Ruffs cost an arm and a leg. Oddly, so do hearts.

Garalt: Wow, either you know just how to pretend the symptoms to queue-jump, or you really do recharge their machines. On the subject of teaching or death, maybe consider option 3?

Christine: I can do Ophelia's mad scene.

Yeah, that's a cheery piece for a memorial service:

'He is dead and gone, lady,
He is dead and gone.
At his head is a patch of green grass,
And at his feet there is a tomb stone.'

Scott: Strippers performing Shakespeare!

Me: YOU, stripped, performing Shakespeare.

Scott: The drunken porter, perhaps!

*We'd **all** have to be drunk.*

Marion: Terry, I have no idea how you are in "real life," but your humor and grace through this has been inspirational. I don't want to say I "enjoy" reading your posts because basically it is just bad news on top of worse news, except in some ways it isn't, because you are still here and you never lose your Terry-ness.

Me: What you see is what you get, I'm afraid. No performing required.

Barbara: I'm surprised they didn't go for a left ventricular assist device. That's kind of like heart surgery, yes, but that would be like a bridge for the transplant.

Me: They say they can't really do that with this rare amyloid thing I have.
Cindi: As much as Shakespeare and strippers would make for an unforgettable send off, I'm praying your wait for a new heart won't be long.

Shylock's working on getting me one as we speak.

Julie: I don't want to help Janet make breakaway farthingales.

The breakaway corsets would be harder to do.

Robin: Um, is this the point where I tell you that I've based a secondary character off you (though I don't know you truly, deeply?) And, like, are the strippers taking it off to Bach and reciting Shakespeare while they do?

*Not Bach, no. This **actual** Elizabethan song will do.*

Will you buy a fine dog?
by Thomas Morley, 1600

'Will you buy a fine dog, with a hole in its head?
With a dildo, with a dildo, dildo, with a dildo, dildo, dildo;
muffs, cuffs, ribatos, and fine sisters' thread.
With a dildo, with a dildo, dildo, with a dildo, dildo;
I stand not on points, pins, periwigs, combs, glasses,
Gloves, garters, girdles, busks, for the brisk lasses;
But I have other dainty, dainty tricks,
Sleek stones and potting sticks.
With a dildo, dildo, dildo, diddle diddle dildo, with a diddle, diddle,
And for a need my pretty, pretty, pretty pods
Amber, civet, and musk cods
With a dildo, with a diddle diddle dildo,
with a diddle, diddle, diddle, diddle, diddle, diddle, diddle, diddle dildo,
with a dildo, diddle, diddle, diddle, diddle, diddle, diddle dildo.'

Yeah, you counted right. This is a 20-dildo book. Wholesome fun for the whole family.

Which reminds me that my basset hound once came home with one. Nobody ever showed up to claim it. Not joking.

Sarah: We did have a traveling pole for *The Tempest* last year...how big is your hospital room?

Me: About 15 X 20. You'll have to work around about $200,000 worth of cutting-edge medical equipment.

Phlebotomist came in at 3:30 in the flipping morning to draw blood. I was actually sleeping, which is a hospital miracle. I feel the jab and

then hear, "Oops! How did that happen? Sorry, I have to stick you again."

Hopefully the Transplant Team is more on the ball.

FYI, a phlebotomist jabs you with a needle and takes your blood. That's all they do, day in and day out. So one would expect a certain amount of precision. I need to do this in my classroom: "Oops! How did that happen? Sorry, I have to flunk you again."

Maria: Didn't even buy you a drink!

*For all I know, Bloody Mary was draining me to **get** a drink.*

Theresa: It was the best of times, it was the worst of times ..." Oh, who are we kidding...lol

Judith: During one of my hospital stays, a new tech came to draw blood at the witching hour — 3:30 a.m. As he fumbled around with the tray and such, he apologized and announced he would have to turn on the light. I assured him I would much rather he turn on the light before he stuck me with the huge needle he had, than do it in the dark.

Me: Mine all do the blood draws in the dark.

You know, I'm a transplant to Colorado from Illinois, but this is taking the metaphor a bit too far.

I was just told that if I ask the actual transplant surgical team nicely, I might get a selfie with my old heart. #notjoking

Me: After all, I already showed my brain scan to my students.

Liana: You should have them video the whole thing!

I imagine they would, since this is a teaching hospital and I'm a rarity.

Ana: Facebook Live!

Me: I could pre-record comic narration to go over it.

Me: With Benny Hill theme music.

Liana: Or Laurel and Hardy music.

Mark: Gonna keep it in a jar and name him?

Me: Can't keep it. They use them for research, especially mine with the weird rare disease they need to know more about.

Melanie: You're a research project!

There will probably be an 800-slide PowerPoint presentation about me, with Mannheim Steamroller music and a laser light show.

Virginia: Well, it's all about who you know in there to get anything allowed. OR is just their everyday office.

Me: My cardiologist RUNS the transplant center, so...

Tim: I have a pic of the new heart but never ended up getting a pic of the old heart.

This hospital averages a heart transplant every week, so I guess I don't have to worry about the surgeons skills being rusty.

Me: They've done 500 of them.

Maria: Ah, good. Nice to know they like to keep their hand in.

Helen: Or two.

Oh, there's a lot more than 2 hands in there at a time. The videos look like somebody dropped a $100 bill in the patient's chest cavity.

Scott: Yes, you want experienced cardio warriors on this. You don't need a heart-dazed knight.

I trust that you know the way to the exit?

Day 5 of the Magical Mystery Tour.
Or Day 1 of the 'Whose Heart Will He Get?' vigil.

Kristi: It is going to be a long process, but you will get there! Thinking of you daily. My daughter is on day 48 of a hospital stay with her pregnancy. Hoping she goes 5 more weeks. She has video games, crocheting, reading to keep her busy. Do you knit?!

Me: No, but I have 2 novels to finish writing and 2 more to edit. Plus, 2 stories have to go out to the next Rocky Mountain Fiction Writers anthology.

If I'd had to stay in that hospital for 10 weeks, you'd have been reading headlines on the national news like "Deranged patient slays 74 in Colorado medical center."

"But he seemed so nice,' says lucky survivor."

My stepdaughter was driving past motorcyclists without helmets and considered a little surprise swerve, just to increase the donor pool. #that'sfamilyloyaltyforyou.

Janet: But first asking their blood type.

Ana: And if they're signed up as a donor.

Alaena: And actually they were cyclists. Your peeps.

Me: You monsters.

Alaena: Sticking to 6-foot mid-adult male bicyclists. We got plenty around my house. We'll just drive around and ask their blood types. Find the right one and have Mom "slip" while driving. (cataracts, didn't see him). Heart availability solved. **I'm going to Hell; we'll pad that handbasket**

Erin: Must cull the MAMIL population for the growth of the species (Middle Aged Male in Lycra)

Me: I'm elderly now, so back off. #EMIL

And my ass looks spectacular in Lycra, I'll have you know.

Erin: But don't you want a "young buck heart", preferably one already accustomed to biking long distances? I'm only suggesting the right fit for ya.

Looks like this place may be more *Grey's Anatomy* than I thought. There are six — SIX — pregnant cardiology nurses on this floor.

Julia: Well, they can't blame you. You haven't been there long enough.

Sarah: Don't drink the water!

Probably a 'heart-on' joke here someplace, but I'm taking the high road for once.

The infectious diseases doctor was here telling me about all of the things I won't be allowed to do once I'm immune-suppressed. And at least one good thing is coming from all of this lunacy.

I never have to pick up dog poop again.

Me: You're on the hook here, honeybunch. I have a doctor's note.

Tina: Remember this when the worst is over and he's healthy enough to exact revenge!

Jim: You'll need to replace your bassets with "low-emission" dogs.

Maria: Not even wearing gloves?

Me: Nope.

Bren: Did you already get your shingles vaccine? Presuming you had chicken pox and not the chicken pox vaccine, it now resides in your spine and waits until your immunity is low before it works its way out through your muscles and becomes a rash. The thing is, as it works its way through your muscles, you swear you're being shivved in the back/side/kidneys. Shingles is, in my opinion, the number one reason for vaccinating children against chicken pox. The vaccination is a mild strain that does not return as shingles when you're older or immune-compromised.

Me: They're giving me that and a gazillion others.

Tim: No changing kitty litter.

Not a cat fancier by any stretch of the imagination, so that's not a concern. Plus, Janet's allergic to the furry little demons.

This is the protein scaffold that remains after a heart has had all of its cells removed. Called a "ghost heart," this scaffold can then be injected with hundreds of millions of blood or bone-marrow stem cells from the transplant recipient, which lowers the chance of rejection. This procedure has been conducted in pigs and rodents thus far and shows promising results. (photo 24)

Who the hell got a grant to do heart transplants on rodents? And what does he/she have for dinner table conversation at the end of the day? "Bad day today. The beaver didn't make it."

And aren't all transplanted hearts 'ghost' hearts, really?

And now we're back to 3 heparin shots a day (to prevent blood clots), plus at least 1 daily blood test. And I'm about to get a gazillion vaccinations to make up for having my immune system nuked later. Needles, needles, needles…more than if I were diabetic.

Little did I know that after the surgery they'd treat me like a diabetic and finger-stick me 4 or 5 times a day. That got really old really fast. If I actually got diabetes, I'd whine more than a French vineyard.

4/5/19
If I hang garlic on my bed rail, will that keep the Brides of Dracula from taking my blood at 3:30 a.m. every night?

Janet: Is that why I get UC Health updates on the phone all night?

Me: Yep.

We have the UC Health app on all of our electronic doohickeys. One part of it records your tests in real time as the hospital gets them. It pings every time. As I write this, there are several hundred test results there.

And it makes me indescribably happy that my spell-checker actually flagged 'doohickeys' and corrected the spelling.

Given what's soon to happen, I should change my religious affiliation to 'Aztec.'

Scott: I've always said that you put your heart into everything you do.

Take my heart out of everything, you mean.

Stephanie: Scott, though you meant this as a joke (and I laughed) there is great truth in your words.

Me: For a brief moment on the operating table, I'll literally be heartless.

Liana: According to your students, it won't be the first time, however.

Hey, I'm brutal, but I'm fair.

Cerene: You should get a video of the surgeon saying, "Kali Ma Shakti de!" as they change 'em out.

Me: And then Harrison Ford starts massacring the entire surgical team.

Jacqueline: I think that only works if they use an obsidian knife.

Tinney: Points for style, Terry, throughout this whole ordeal.

Danica: If I ever have a significant health challenge, I hope I do it with your amazing attitude!

This is scoring that handicapped parking sticker the hard way.

But since my condition won't be visible, I'd still have to fake a limp to keep the parking lot 'Are you really handicapped?' Nazis at bay. What is it with those people? They must be the same ones who drive around their housing developments measuring other people's fence heights.

The next test they do on me here will be the 100th since midnight Sunday when I arrived.

Me: About 20 a day.

Mark: At least you're getting your money's worth.

Mark: What, do they think you've suddenly been replaced with a clone? The 'mirror-universe Terry Kroenung'?

Julie: The evil Terry would not have a beard.

Me: They're ALL evil Terry!

I just managed to get the top doc here to order a Do Not Disturb for me, so no more nighttime venous stabbings.

Another moment of spectacular naivete.

Yep. It's official. Level 3. This is Day 1 of the countdown. (photo 25)

Janet: That must mean the insurance finally agreed?

Me: Yep. They won't list you otherwise.

Linda: Sure as hell not like this in Canada. We are on the list, period, rich or poor, or whatever. What f**king difference does the insurance make? Need a heart in Canada? NO MONEY REQUIRED!!! This is appalling. Shame on the American government for not caring!

Alaena: Reading the listing/transplant requirements was eye opening. They talk about financial ability to pay every couple of paragraphs and if they think your situation is in any way not financially viable long term, they won't list.

Barbara: Level III? I couldn't read the print on the sheet, so I'm wondering does that mean you get to wait at home?

Me: No, because the hospital insisting I'm too sick to leave puts me higher than I otherwise would be.

Maria: Shouldn't being a teacher put you at the top of list because karma points?

Me: In a sane and sensible world, yes.

Especially considering the dire teacher shortage. I had an administrator tell me during my evaluation that it didn't much matter how bad I was, he had nobody to replace me. Not sure how much of that was a joke.

Maria: Though in a sane sensible world it wouldn't be up to insurance to put you on the damn list.

Tina: Seems unreal until you see it in writing…with instructions, too.

Maria: It's actually a very structured process. My mother-in-law had a liver transplant last year, and it's like a space mission. You have a team. You have a timeline. When the transplant becomes available, they call you THAT MOMENT, you drop everything and go. In her case, she was at home, not at the hospital, but otherwise, yeah.

Jesus, Mary, and Joseph…it took 2 nurses 3 tries to put the new IV in. Those aren't like the wimpy little blood draws. They freaking hurt. But the old ones had to come out. One went bad and inflamed my arm. The other was a ginormous arterial needle put in by the ablation team while I was sedated (thank Odin). It hurt to push anything through it.

I'm so covered in bruises and gouges now that if I was anywhere but a hospital, someone would call in an abuse report. Just another

hot Friday night in paradise.

And those 2 bad IV sites are still messed up as I type this 4 months later. They feel like solid leather tubes. My Transplant Team looked at them, shrugged, and said, "Oh, yeah. Thromboses. Those can take months and months to go away."

Me: "Local man escapes abductors. Film at 11."

Christine: When I came out of having brain surgery, I had six IV ports in me...front and back of both my hands (4), one in my neck, and one in my left ankle. I found weird tape marks after that for a couple of weeks.

Me: That's what the transplant will give me.

It turned out to be 3 arm/hand lines and 1 in the neck. And 9 post-op drainage tubes. I looked like aliens were trying to clone a captive human.

Christine: When Hope had Squidgie I was surprised to learn that Longs Peak likes to have the paramedics do IV's if they're available, because they tend to do them more frequently out in the field and so are better at them.

Kelly: Well, they're not supposed to make you feel worse.

Me: Oh, this will get worse before it gets better. Google 'heart transplant recovery room images.'

Kelly: You need to quit looking stuff up! You're gonna be on anxiety meds if you aren't already.

Maria: Holy cow, are they using those oil pipelines they use for blood donors?

No, it just feels like they are.

Jim: 'Not so deep as a well nor as wide as a church door...'

4/6/19
That Do Not Disturb order wasn't worth the pixels it was printed in. 3:20 a.m., there they were again, drawing blood and making me get

out of bed to check my flipping weight. I'm not gonna weigh more or less at 7 a.m., ladies.

Marisa: Geez. why are they testing so late/early?

Me: They want all the tests done by the time doctors arrive on their rounds.

Julia: I think nurses train at the same place as waiters who ask you how everything is as soon as you get your mouth full.

And dentists who want to ask you about your life with two fists halfway down to your liver.

Kelly: Why are they taking blood every day?

Hey, who **wouldn't** *want a piece of this?*

Me: They have to make sure my systems don't degrade, because you have to be healthy enough to survive this monstrous surgery.

Deborah: All that information and lab results must be completed before the physicians start showing up on the floor to do their rounds. Physicians do hospital rounds first thing in the morning, then they return to their offices, where the see more patients, and after hours they may do another set of hospital rounds, to follow up on the more critical patients. It's a pain to be awakened so early in the morning, and patients never really get good sleep while hospitalized. But there really is a good reason for the craziness. Hope this helps a little.

Oh, sure, that's what they **tell** *you…*

Bill: My hospital bed at Evergreen also records my weight. They were concerned when I suddenly put on seven pounds—and lost it once I put my Surface on the bedside table. Get well. Hope they find the heart of a fighter for you.

Virginia: I figured it wouldn't. Shifts always claim that they missed the notice.

Just to show you how random this amyloidosis thing is, I just walked a mile, 5 laps around this floor, without any problems. Pulse briefly at 122, but mostly around 100. Pretty lame for a 22:00 mile, but I AM getting a freaking heart transplant, after all.

Yesterday afternoon I barely got through a single lap. Pulse spiked to tachycardia level, 151, and the alarms went off. Felt crappy. Go figure.

I figure there are tiny cardiac gremlins in there, randomly pulling levers and stomping on pedals, cackling in manic glee.

Just got yelled at by the charge nurse for daring to walk without permission. Apparently my low-fall-risk status has to be renewed by her every morning. #youaren'tthebossofme!

Beth: #yessheisthebossofyoufornow

Me: What's she gonna do, kill me?

Liana: She could insert another IV line v-e-r-y painfully if you don't behave.

This is my first full day of watching the news for word of a local multi-fatality highway pileup resulting in lots of young, healthy people on life support. #I'mgoingtohell

They just pushed the first drip through the new IV, and it already hurts like hell. WTF???

Me: Didn't hurt till she flushed it with saline.

Janet: Ouch. Salt in the wound?

Bonnie: What are they giving you?

Me: They were just replacing an old bad one. I have to have one, in case there's an emergency.

Bonnie: Ask for a PICC line; all meds can be given and labs can be drawn through one. Surprised they didn't put one in already.

Me: They're doing blood draws through the IV now. Not a fan of a PICC line again unless everything else fails.

Eventually they just treated the scary neck port like a PICC line.

Shingles shot yesterday, hurts like a hammer blow from Thor today. Just got a pneumonia shot in the other arm, expecting the same later. #runningoutofarms

Janet: Your arms are so skinny anyway.

Me: This is true.

Barbara: Why the shingles shot?

Me: I have to be inoculated against a ton of potentially dangerous things, because my immune system will be shot. In my case, shingles could wreck most of your organs and kill you.

Maria: That's to be expected. Shingles shots suck. Oooh, what a marvelous tongue twister! You could amuse yourself while saying it five times faster after the pain meds kick in.

If Peter Piper picked a peck of PICC lines...

Had a heart offered already, but they decided it was too small, plus they don't like to put female hearts in guys. Underpowered.

Carrie: Oh, wow, this is so stressful, I can't imagine!

Me: Imagine a prison with a view of the mountains where you pay THEM $25K a day to jab you with needles and to yank your beating heart out like an Aztec sacrifice. But with decent food, actually.

Menu suggestion: Superior Vena Cavatappi.

Maria: Ok, that's new. I didn't know that.

Me: I didn't either, until the morning horde of MD's strolled through.

Cheri: Whoa! I had no idea they were different sizes and horsepower. The human body is strange. Here's hoping they get you one with a souped-up engine. Maybe a 70's muscle car type?

Probably end up with Chitty-Chitty bang-Bang.

The Infectious Diseases doctor from India was here, and all she did was grill me about her adopting a rescue basset hound.

Maria: Finally! We are talking about something relevant!

Jim: Sounds like you should charge her for that visit.

Good idea. I'll invoice her for $1.8 million and break even on all of this.

Marti: If she wanted you to adopt a rescue dog then she must think you are gonna be around for a while to take care of a dog! That's encouraging and good news!

Me: No, SHE wants a dog.

Not sure I sold the product well, though, telling her about the drool, the hound funk, the shedding, and being a bond-slave to a 12-inch-high dictator.

Just walked another mile in the hall, average pulse 104, though it briefly spiked to 144. Only a 23:30 pace, but the nurses act like I'm Captain America, since nobody else here in the Cardiac ICU can get out of bed. They seem to usually leave feet-first.

Me: I'm going to hold a walk-a-thon, raise some cash to pay for this transplant.

Let's see, that means I only have to walk to Mars and back to raise enough $.

Fiona: Love you so much, Terry. Your saga has been equally amusing me and worrying me for days. There's a book in this, you know!

So everyone keeps saying. Mustn't deny the people what they want, especially if I get to charge them for it.

Alicia: Just shows how tough you are! After the transplant, maybe aim for a marathon.

Not sure that the heart doctors having their morning meeting around a box of donuts sets the proper example for the languishing residents of the Cardiac Intensive Care Unit. Likewise, the box at the nurses' station, too.

My cardiac team is the Crispy Crème of the crop.

Sessha: Maybe they are giving you something to aim for?

Alaena: Did you steal one on your walk? If not, you should.

Me: Good thing I didn't, considering.

I can't have any open, in-common food now. No buffets, salad bars, etc. Finally, a legit reason to avoid Golden Corral…though that's potentially fatal to healthy people, too.

Eric: Maybe now that the transplant's a go for tonight, this would be an opportune time to have one of the donuts? Or for that matter maybe an extra well-marbled porterhouse?

Me: They made me stop eating and drinking. Haven't eaten in 13+ hours already.

Sean: Tell them to brush the crumbs off their scrubs before they lean over you.

Virginia: Typical. At least they don't go out to smoke any more.

On the over-sharing front, I proudly announced to my nurse's

assistant that I had produced the stool sample demanded from on high. She said she'd collect it and send it to the lab. A minute later, she was putting on a hazmat gown, gloves, and mask. #fearsomepoop

Me: Apparently that was for a different patient.

Maria: Wait, WHAT?! Another patient needed your stool sample?

*They transplant everything here (and yes, you **can** transplant that, when someone needs to restart their gut bacteria from scratch). #notjoking*

Me: Transplant tonight. That must've been one HELL of a good stool sample.

Maria: I was just going to say...isn't there a fairy tale about a donkey who could poop gold coins?

With what this is going to cost, I could use a herd of those.

Marti: Did you tell the nurse that shit happens?

I'm pretty sure she was aware, at that point.

To access the photos/videos/links:
www.terrykroenungink.com/246-2/

4) Pardon me, I was using that heart!

April 7-April 16, 2019

Here we go, surgical procedure fans, the actual transplantation part and all of the hilarity that went with it.

Fun fact: removing the heart is called 'explantation.' Probably because calling it 'hacking the old ticker out with buzzsaws and murder-knives' doesn't exactly encourage people to line up to have it done.

We were offered a heart the very day I was put on the list. That was unusual enough. But the donor was a five-foot-tall woman and the Transplant Team passed on it. Too underpowered, they said, for my size and conditioning. Well, you don't drive a Maserati with a VW Beetle motor, do you? Plus, it seems that there's a higher rate of complications (a polite term for 'tragic death after we went and did all of this damned work') when a female heart is put into a guy. That isn't the case the other way around, oddly.

That was Thursday. I had a good heart donated on Friday, only 20 hours after going on the list. Practically a record. 50 hours later, they wheeled me off for the transplant. During those 50 hours, I wasn't allowed the slightest morsel of food and barely any water. Yeah, I was 'hangry' by the time the orderly came to get me.

So in the space of a long weekend, starting about 2 p.m. Friday and going until just after midnight Monday morning, I went from "You know, I really don't feel all that bad, I think I'll walk 2 miles in the hall" (which I did) to "Hey, I woke up from this with a new heart, which I honestly didn't think I'd survive."

From then on it was a week of being tethered to literally a dozen IV pumps, feeding me all manner of stupefyingly-expensive goo to keep the heart going, to keep my body from rejecting it, and to keep at bay the awful side-effects of the first two. The surgery and meds made me temporarily diabetic, so I got to experience the unalloyed giddy fun times of finger sticks and insulin shots (lifetime diabetics, I feel your pain...a little).

Oh, and if you still think this would be a joyous romp for yourself: I was epically constipated for that whole week from the meds, despite the super-strength IV laxatives dumped into me. Whole teams of doctors and nurses kept inquiring about my pooping progress, like it was going to bring world peace if I managed to flush my toilet.

4/7/19
Holy...shit. My transplant happens tonight.

So April 7: second birthday.

Jennifer: Holy shit! For serious?? Will someone be able to update your FB and let us know when you're all clear? Oh, my word. Sending you every last good vibe I can wrangle.

Me: Wife will do that.

Donna: What?????

Me: Yep. First full day on the list. I don't dick around.

Somebody probably figured out that I'm the world's most impatient patient.

Justin: You'll be back to normal in no time, I'm sure, whether or not you are supposed to be back to normal or not. Thoughts are absolutely with you, gonna have to visit my favorite teacher after all this mess is said and done.

'Normal?' Sir, you insult me!

Carrie: Go, go, new heart! I'm rooting for you!!!

Me: 'The Little Organ That Could.'

Old heart: 'The Organ That Couldn't ~~Be~~ Beat.'

Sarah: How long is the surgery?

Me: 4-10 hours. All depends on how things go once they're in there.

"Holy crap! look at all the cobwebs in here. Nurse, hand me that Dustbuster."

Me: About the same as that wretched ablation I had Tuesday, that they clearly could have skipped.

Ended up being almost exactly as long as the ablation. And I felt better after the transplant than after that one.

Maria: The very cool part about this (and I do know this) is that the new organ begins doing its job immediately after they got it sewn into place. It might still be healing, but it is already doing what it's supposed to do.

One would hope that there wouldn't be a 3-day lag time on the heart working. I'd have to think twice about paying the full rate.

Janet O.: Wow, Terry. Prayers coming. Blessings to the person who is giving you a second chance in life. More Shakespeare!

Julia: Also, prayers for the family of the donor. And a thank you to them, also.

Stephanie: Looking forward to meeting the new you...whom I expect to be just like the old you but with an awesome scar.

Awesome ain't the half of it. 9-inch heart scar, 3-inch pacemaker removal, plus 9 drainage tube sites that look like I was shotgunned.

Geoffrey: Best goddamn thoughts!!

Me: Standard SAFD pep talk to surgeons: 'Don't fuck up!'

Society of American Fight Directors. That saying is commonly heard right before a Skills Proficiency Test or as the curtain going up on the show you choreographed.

Christine: That has got to be the best news I've heard in a long time, Terry & Janet. I propose we celebrate your new birthday with those strippers and Shakespeare scenes you mentioned earlier.

Might want to wait on the strippers until the heart vessel stitches heal.

Sheila: I'll be holding you in my virtual heart, so your new heart won't get lonely.

Julie: But I haven't even sent you a card yet. Quit outpacing me.

I can only do that until they yank out the pacemaker.

My late lunch arrived just as he was telling me I couldn't eat or drink now.

This is precisely why hospital victims are called 'patients.'

Diagnosed with the amyloidosis exactly one month ago tomorrow. That may be a record for diagnosis to transplant.

Janet: Geez, you just got listed less than 24 hours ago. I don't know about you but my brain hasn't caught up yet.

You should try it from my end. None of my parts has caught up yet.

Eric: Like the "I'll have what she's having" line from *When Harry Met Sally*— I'll have the insurance he has...

This is the best way to do it. No time to dwell on it at all.

Not sure *300* is the movie I want to watch while waiting for my heart transplant.

Me: *Moulin Rouge* is my other choice. Not much better.

Maria: Well, at least you can sing along with *Moulin Rouge*...and it's got a much better selection of corsets and fishnet stockings. Just saying.

So does 'The Rocky Horror Picture Show,' but that would be an even worse choice, considering.

Though I'd pay top dollar to see Gerard Butler in fishnets and spike heels.

Elise: Avoid *Royal Hunt of the Sun,* too.

For the uninitiated: that's a movie about Montezuma and the Aztecs.

David: Maybe *Fantastic Voyage?*

Believe me, I'd prefer a nano-sub and a tiny laser to what's about to happen.

Me: I found a *Twilight Zone* marathon. That's the ticket.

Christine: Find someone with a copy of Cosby's classic "The Chicken Heart".

He got that from a real old-time radio show in the 30's.

Amber: Better than *Temple of Doom.*

Scott: Gotta be *Titanic.* Okay, awful movie, but this is the day for "My Heart Will Go On."

"Put your hands on me, doc."

Christine: But Scott, I thought the whole point of this exercise is that Terry's old, protein-encrusted heart will not go on.

Serge: Joseph Schildkraut in "The Tell-Tale Heart"?

They can bury my old one under the floorboards if they want.

It would seem that my transplant surgeon is the envy of all of the other transplant surgeons here. #gettingmymoney'sworth

Tim: Same for me. He's also my regular cardiologist and has done most of my post-transplant biopsies.

Christine: Curious, what do they biopsy post-transplant?

They run a probe through your jugular vein and scrape cells off of the inside of your right atrium. It's as much fun as it sounds.

Tim: They are checking for rejection. Since rejection is asymptomatic, they do biopsies. Weekly at first. Then every other week. Then every 4-6 weeks. Eventually the goal is annually with a blood test called Allomap in between.

Maybe I can find a showing of *'The Merchant of Venice'* before the transplant.

"If you prick us, do we not bleed?"

Midnight. No word yet on the heart. Just sitting here waiting.

And I kept waiting. It was a heart day's night.

Julia: Do you know if it's local or if they have to fly it in?

Me: They didn't say.

Tim: Mine was delayed a few hours because they were harvesting other organs and the heart needs to go last.

Me: That's what's happening here.

Christine: Sounds like you will not be the only one receiving a new beginning tonight.

Tim: Each donor can donate up to 8 organs.

Ana: Wasn't there a 4-hour window for a heart?

Me: That clock doesn't start until they remove it and begin transport.

Yikes, the hepatitis A/B shot hurts going in. Good thing that's not a weekly occurrence. I'm guessing it's nothing to having your sternum bisected with a circular saw, though. #it'sallrelative

Christine: Are these shots going to have time to take effect before the big event?

Me: Apparently.

Or maybe it was just the nurses' idea of a hilarious prank. "For real, he believes that shingles is the actual serious name of a disease. Can you believe the gullibility of some people?"

Shingles sounds like what you get after you've been roofied at a rave.

4/7/19
7:45 a.m. No transplant yet. Still waiting. Looks like they may be harvesting the other organs first, to help the maximum number of people. Hearts go last, as they support everything else.

Me: Awake half the night, because every voice or footstep got interpreted as "here they are."

Sort of the way it goes down on Death Row, I imagine.

Barbara: I would think that the organ has to be transplanted quickly after harvesting.

Around 4 hours to get it out, transported, and put in, or the cells start dying.

Kate: I expect after this long night of waiting, you're ready to cut someone yourself.

Wisely, I limited myself to cutting remarks.

Rebecca: Thinking of you, try to be patient.

Donna: Umm…he is a patient.

Maria: Hang in there, bud! We are almost there! Spread your ribs and think of Shakespeare!

Me: After noon now, they say. #stillnofood

(Jim P.): So - in the "my life isn't THAT bad" category, while I'm feeling mopey about my normal list of Sunday chores, I know that a friend is still waiting for the heart transplant that was supposed to start last night. Blessings and peace and patience for you, Terry, and Janet, and may the surgical team be well-rested.

Me: Yeah, I won't be able to complain about any other damned thing imaginable after this.

Oh, yes, I can. Watch and learn, young paduan.

Docs say they're about to transport my new heart. Surgery should be early afternoon.

But, Dear Reader, I was cruelly deceived.

Paula: Prayers for good health. If it means anything, my uncle had a heart transplant 30 years ago, and is out on the golf course today. Good luck. They've gotten much better.

Pierre: If they save the old one, I can make you a Christmas Organament.

Me: Sorry. My disease is so rare that they're planning to slice it up and do experiments on it. Gotta get those research grants.

Siobahn: Sending positive vibes (and a little racy giggle), Terry. **(Photo 26)**

Daniel: See if they can let you keep your old heart. You can keep it in a chest for Pirates of the Caribbean cosplay.

But it's already in a chest.

Regan: Terry, I want to thank you for sharing your journey for your heart. We see news reports and articles about how important it is to become an organ donor — and sometimes we hear of a success. But I can't think of a time someone shared their journey to get there — to get that, as you put it yesterday, their second birthday. It takes great courage to live day to day knowing you need help — an organ. It takes even more courage to share the way there with people. So thank you for taking the time and giving the gift of your journey. Heartfelt prayers as you go forward.

Just had a doctor say that I was on shockingly few medications for someone about to get a heart transplant.

Adam: Presumably, a good thing as less clashes between them?

Me: It's a good thing because that means I'm crazy healthy otherwise.

Janet always says that I'm the world's sickest healthy person.

One 2-hour round of anti-rejection meds infused, and round 2 about to start.

Dai: I wish I could have given those to some of the women I've met!

*Having experienced them, it **so** wouldn't get you laid.*

You know, I've always been into recycling, but this may be a bridge too far.

Me: "Hearts in the blue bin, livers in the green bin..."

Erin: My husband, the son of a cardiac nurse (which here in the NHS means she's the one who literally does everything but the transplant itself), groaned when I told him this remark. I'm going to send her this comment now. I really do love the sense of humor right now.

Tim: My sister sent me a t-shirt with the recycle symbol with a heart inside with the words "contains recycled parts."

I have that same shirt now, because, of course, I do.

Perry: They should get you a playlist:
"Anyone Who Had a Heart" - Cilla Black
"The Heart's Filthy Lesson"- David Bowie
"My Heart will Go On" - Celine Dion

Wade: I heard one of the Rockerfellers had 8 heart transplants. I think he finally passed on recently.

Don't ever dare to tell me that you can't game this supposedly neutral system.

Alas for our outrage, that proved to be an urban myth, based on a parody story attacking the 1%.

I KNEW this was a real movie. I recall seeing it.

***Return to Me* (2000). Starring David Duchovny, Minnie Driver. "A man, who falls in love with the woman who received his wife's heart, must decide which woman it is who holds his heart." (link #3)**

Better than that other famous transplant flick, 'Mad Love' (1935), where surgeon Peter Lorre loses his hands and is transplanted with those of a knife murderer. The hands take over and hilarity ensues.

Erin: I actually really like this movie. It's sweet.

Seemed like it was just a sneaky way to justify Duchovny putting his hand on Minnie's chest. "Hey, it's a legit plot point!"

Officially-recognized transplant-related observances for this date:

World Health Day
National Beer Day

Somebody didn't think that through. Though Ben Franklin did say, "Beer is proof that God loves us and wants us to be happy."

Heart transplant humor. Saw a cartoon where the transplant surgeon had a heart in each hand and asked, "Now the old one's in my right hand and the donor's is in the left...right?"

Curtis: We all know **your** heart's in the right place.

Is it, though…really?

Saw another cartoon where the heart was on the floor and the doc hollered, "Five second rule!"

1:30 pm and still waiting for the transplant surgery. Nobody here has any info.

Curtis: Hopefully they haven't given it to someone else by mistake.

Kind of hoping they already stamped a bar-code on it. They did it to me. #notjokingmuch

Me: 24 hours since I was notified. 28+ since I was allowed to eat.

They'll come to take me to pre-op and all they'll find is vultures circling over bones.

Tim: I was thinking about this. Hopefully the heart arrives soon.

Maybe the heart took a wrong turn at Albuquerque.

It's now been longer waiting for the transplant surgery after notification of a heart than the time I was ON the list.

The anesthesiology resident had me sign the release for the industrial-strength sleepy-time meds, so it shouldn't be too much longer (one would think).

So I can't claim to be 'woke.'

3 p.m. They just came in and said the heart is STILL in the donor in New Mexico, as all of the other organs haven't been removed. It could every late tonight before anything hearty actually happens. #losingsenseofhumor

Michael: At least they haven't taken your old one out already.

Harriet: Okay, so if it's coming from New Mexico, do we need to start green chile therapy so you'll accept it?

Can't eat peppers because of the reflux, so that would be a problem.

Surgeon just came in (David Fullerton). Older than me, Mr. Cool, full business suit and tie, a doctor straight out of central casting. He expects to be rolling on this transplant business in a couple of hours.

Liana: Let's all shower Terry with hearts to let him know we're going to be with him 'in heart' in the operating room and recovery! I'll go first.

"Let's all shower with Terry" would've been a bigger morale-booster.

(Donna): T minus 2 hours & counting...Terry Kroenung gets his new ticker. Prayers should be flowing...please.

Andrea: It occurs to me that 'Krönung' in German means "coronation". Lovely to note that the Italian word for heart is coro. Lots of sovereign energy surrounds you!

It's also the biggest brand of coffee in Germany, though I've seen no royalties so far.

4:30 p.m. They're taking me to the OR for the transplant, kids. Catch you on the flip side.

Me: Janet will be posting updates here until I'm back in the loop, which will be a while.

Russ: I dedicated my yoga practice to you today, Terry.

The Reclined Hero pose, I hope.

(Janet; 5:35 pm) Terry has been prepped and is on the way to OR. It will take 4 to 5 hours minimum. Could take up to 8 hours. Fingers crossed, praise to all the deities including Kali and the Aztec heart

gods. A nod to the Tin Man, and to *Iron Man*, which was on Terry's TV just as they wheeled him out, I kid you not.

Nothing wrong with me that an oil can, arc reactor, and rousing musical numbers can't fix.

Terry S.: Oz never did give nothing to the Tin Man that he didn't already have. He's got plenty of it...and is going to get more!

Pay no attention to that man behind the curtain...he's just the anesthesiologist.

Shannon: Tin Man power!

I need a testimonial heart clock...and an axe.

Laura: I'll take the *Iron Man* movie to be a good sign! Sending all my best up to those who may be listening!

(Janet; 6:30 pm) They started the actual operation about 20 minutes ago.

Max: I wanna see the selfie with the original.

Alas, it was not to be. Those selfish @#$! physicians Bogarted it.

(Janet): They are still working.

Christine: Okay, thank you, Janet. How are you holding up?

Janet: Beyond tired. Sitting in a little waiting room. At least the bunch of noisy teens left.

*I imported those so I'd have my normal classroom environment. It **is** a teaching hospital.*

(Janet; 10:32 pm) Getting closer. Maybe an hour and half or two.

Christine: That's great news, it means the whole thing will take around 5 hours which suggests everything is going as expected!!!

I got to sleep through it all. Poor Janet was a nervous wreck.

(Janet; 11:24 pm) Doctor just called and they are closing him up now. In about another hour and a half they will move him to recovery and I can see him. New heart is working fine.

♫ Zippity-doo-da, zippity-day!

AE: Oh, wow!!! What great news!!!! Love to EVERYONE involved, you guys, the surgeons and staff and blessings to the donor family. There is so much love surrounding him right now — I can feel it!

Janet: Thank you all for the support. Stage one of the process is done! Now to watch for rejection and bleeding. Terry will hurt like hell and he doesn't do well with pain.

Hey! I resent that! I'm a paragon of stoic courage and – ow! Paper cut! Ooohh!

Christine: Here's hoping that he realizes the pain beats the alternative and that he doesn't get too cranky with you or the nursing staff.

Janet: I told him that already. He knows, but he's still going to be a royal pain.

Royal, huh? I'm Count Cardiac!

Karen: Hugs & kisses to you both. Guess that kind of close contact stuff will be off the table for the foreseeable future, but I am so glad you are onto the next stage: A grand entrance cometh and all shall be well(er).

Cindi: You must be exhausted, Janet. I know Terry relies on you so much. I hope you have people you can lean on through all of this. Thank you for the updates.

Sheila: It has been an amazing experience thus far with messages from the hospital and sardonic observations along the way. Thank you for the update.

4/8/19
(Janet; 12:52 am) A very tired doctor just came out to tell me that they moved Terry to recovery and that in about an hour they will let me see him. He will be out for some time. I have only had a few naps in the chair since Friday night, so when he looks stable later this morning, I'm going to crash with the dog at Alaena's house. I've been in the same clothes and need a shower and toothpaste, too. But cheers to a very respected and experienced surgeon!

Garalt: Our best wishes for Terry's recovery, and soothing Perry Como Muzak wallpaper for you. Love from Dublin.

Rebecca: Such good news , I can't wait to see the snarky posts in a week or so.

A week? You poor, innocent child.

(Janet; 2:44 am) I'm in recovery with Terry. He's already starting to wake up. They will remove the breathing tube soon.

And that couldn't happen too soon. They could use those things for 'enhanced interrogation.'

(Dean): Very happy for Terry Kroenung who received a new heart last night and is recovering well. Be an organ donor. Save a life.

Sean: I'm looking for a brain transplant.

Me, too, but I'm not letting them anywhere near my groin.

Toni: You certainly don't need anything when you're gone!

(Janet; 7:51 am) Awake! (photo 27)

Janet: They didn't take a picture with the old heart, but he has a 19-year-old new heart.

Veronica: All of his pictures are with his old heart.

Strictly true, I suppose.

Treva: Changes the meaning of "to be young at heart."

Maria: Vintage car — brand new engine. Get to it, man!

Julie: This does not entitle you to blame childishness on your new heart. Get well, my friend.

No, I blame my childishness on that alien abduction I don't like to talk about.

David: Takes a licking and keeps on ticking!

And for you infants under 50, that was the tag line of old Timex watch commercials, where they'd do unspeakable things to their timepieces, like attach them to the propellers of outboard motors.

(Janet; 8:11 am) Terry is still on the ventilator and they are working to get him off.

Rebecca: You realize, he probably won't remember any of this.

Tim: True. I remembered things that didn't happen and forgot things that did. It was that way for a couple of days for me.

(Jim P.): Terry woke up this Monday morning with a heart decades younger than the rest of his body. Seems like an extreme approach for dealing with Mondays, but y'know, you do what you gotta do...

42 years younger, and it always will be.

(Ana): Had to renew my driver's license today online. Of course I selected to remain an organ/tissue donor! My friend Terry Kroenung

just received his new heart last night from a 19yo in New Mexico. Sounds like other organs went to other people as well. #BeAnOrganDonor ! #SaveALife

Mary: Right in the gut, listening to my 19-year-old talking about how he's a donor. Whew!

Ana: And was talking with a friend today: as we move towards autonomous vehicles, there will be less crashes, so less fatalities, so less organ donors. Hopefully, the science steps up to mass produce organs in the lab from stem cells or something.

They're already doing that.

Susan: Just read it's moving toward assumed consent.

Ana: That would be better for first responders, I would imagine.

(Janet; 10:34 am) Terry is in a different wing and different room of the hospital. If you sent cards or packages to the other room's address, we are making arrangements with the other charge nurse to either send them down here or go pick them up. If you haven't, send cards and want to, wait till he gets a permanent room.

It took weeks and weeks to get all of the lost mail.

Somebody swiped my heart and replaced it with a duplicate, like Indiana Jones did with that golden idol. (Photo 28)

Dave: They weren't being literal when they asked you to get it off your chest. Nice to see you, eyes open, channeling Munch!

Janet: Respiration tube is out and Terry is talking again!

The stuff of nightmares. Be afraid…be very afraid.

Mark: Uh-oh!

Russell: Let's hope it's an end to the heartache and the thousand (un)natural shocks...

Didn't immediately end the heartache, but haven't been shocked since, so...win.

Maria: YIKES! That is quite a Christmas tree of an IV stand you've got there!

♫ *"Have yourself a merry little transplant...may your heart be right..."*

Mark: Eeyore and Tigger? Got to be...Tiggers always bounce...

Kristi: Glad to see your tube out and able to talk again! Your color does look better, even Eeyore seems happy!

I went from pasty and gray to merely pasty.

Garalt: This post is on repeat on my FB timeline. How do you get that exposure without actually paying them?

By paying 1.8 million for a heart transplant, that's how. #justgivezuckerberghis$

♫ I'm baaack!

Cheri: No club dancing on tables, now!

Awww, mom, you never let me have any fun.

Andrea: Vrrooommmm!! Incredible!!

Cheri: Hope they are finally letting you eat something!!

Hannah: Oh Terry, you are a trouper! Well done! An age to fall in love!

Matthew: ♫ "Fairy tales can come true, it can happen to you...."

Tim: Great to hear from you. The worst part for me was getting the respirator removed. The rest is easy as pie.

Removing the respirator was a breeze. One hard cough and spit out the accumulated goo. Having it in while waiting for them to all agree when to pluck it out was…not.

Garalt: We'll put the Shakespearean Stripper festival on hold for another 40 years.

Oh, don't put yourself out on my account. If they're already available…

Bill: Let's hear it for those who checked YES on the organ donor question on their driver's license. I'm so glad you got to give life to another person's young heart.

Maria: Oh dear…back on Facebook…with all those pain meds. Are there any adults supervising?

Absolutely not. And I'd ignore them if they were.

AE: Oh yeah — I can tell by this post you are baaaack! Just don't do the Ferrari thing too soon. And doubt you're a Studebaker — maybe a 57 'Chevy — those are classic cars.

Me: I'm a 1958, the same year as the Edsel.

Cindi: !!Yay for modern medicine and blessings to the donor's family. Having been in the donor's shoes at the young age of 31, we felt that donating James' heart and other organs helped comfort us during such a difficult time. I'm really glad that you didn't have to wait a long time!! Heal well.

Mark: We should still get strippers anyway…but we should probably wait until you're a little stronger…

You sound completely selfless about those strippers.

Mark: Whew! Now I don't have to read the "dead parrot" bit at your funeral. Wasn't looking forward to that.

I prefer kippin' on my back. As if I had any choice in a hospital bed with 347 IV lines in me. #piningforthefjords

Perry: Soon you'll be shagging anything longer than it is wide, demanding drugs, and throwing tantrums in between bouts of suicidal depression. Then you'll be all guacamole dip and gender reassignment surgery. Well done.

You sure know how to have a good time.

Katherine: So, basically, you're immortal!!! Yay.

Cindi: You really are Iron Man!

Tina: Be careful not to chase Janet around too much — the legs are YOUR age!

Me: Yeah, but hers are five years older.

Peter: Gad — Remember the Christian Barnard business in '67? Now this isn't even considered rare — The times in which we live, eh?

Sitting in a chair the same day as the heart transplant! (photo 29)

Rebecca: You will be home soon, if you keep this up.

Janet: Here he is, my very own Captain Jean-Luc Picard sitting in his command chair with a new heart. Make it so!

Engage!

Serge: Remember the *Star Trek: The Next Generation* episode where we found that Jean-Luc had an artificial heart, and he took a shuttle to a place where he could get a living one?

I could've used a shuttle, instead of driving an hour each way for every biopsy, etc.

Jim: I dunno — I'm thinking that many tubes, it's Locutus of Borg, not Picard. Time for a daring and highly unorthodox rescue...

Serge: Has Alice Krige been seen around the facilities?

She played the Borg Queen on Star Trek. There, I saved you a trip to Google.

Dai: You're already more energetic than I! Bastard.

Debbie: WHAT!!!! OH, MY GOD, your wife has a young buck to keep up with now. Seriously, I can't believe what modern medicine can do. I'm beyond ecstatic for you, Terry!!!! Hmm, sending hubby for a medical...

David: And tomorrow, the dance marathon?

Spastic old white-guy dancing? Nobody wants to see that.

CS: Those really are outstanding socks.

Garalt: No cycling for at least 24 hours.

Well, I already REcycled.

Perry: I preferred the acoustic Terry to the electric one. Do you have an effects pedal? and a nice Vox AC30? This is more "Into the Black" than "Out of the Blue."

My socks have a fuzz-wah pedal. Their fuzz makes me slip on the tile floor and I flail my arms and yell, "Wha—-?"

Peter: Unbelievable. To me, it still seems so experimental and futuristic.

Sharon: Why are you turning into Big Bird? You have his legs and his feet. Jean-Luc Big Bird.

♫ *"Can you tell me how to get...how to get to Enterprise Street?"*

4/9/19
Words cannot describe how much it hurts to try to breathe with a sawn-through sternum. But coughing hurts SO much worse. That said, my new teenage heart is ticking away unassisted.

*And sneezing **really** sucks.*

Judith: They used to give heart shaped pillows to hug tightly against your chest before you coughed. Not anymore??

Me: They ran out. Big rolled-up hospital blanket works.

Sharon: Use that cheap plastic breathing gizmo often! It really works!

Mark: Just remember to use your pull rope to sit up or move around. Elbows are a no-no. Day One about done. Another day closer to going home.

What is this pull-rope of which you speak? Never saw one.

Liana: And you're ALIVE to feel the pain! It's only the prelude to the first movement of the rest of your life!

Sheila: Now, let's try to make you laugh. That's even worse, but better in a hurts-so-good kind of way.

Cindi: Yeah, I was thinking of you this morning. My hip was hurting and I thought "This is nothing compared to what Terry is probably feeling." Stay strong.

Sarah: It is very important to listen to movement guidelines. My grandma had a bypass and her sternum did not fully knit, so it would shift. Yeah, I know. Just saying it sends goose flesh up my arms. Get to knitting, sir!

When they yanked the multi-branched breathing tube out and I spewed white goo that looked just like android blood from *Alien*, all I could think was "Face hugger!"

Julia: They didn't hurt your sense of humor.

Fiona: Ewwww! Lol!

Serge: Ian Holm or Lance Henriksen?

Oh, why do we have to choose?

John: If we check your DNA, are we going to find a Weyland-Yutani imprint there someplace?

The greedy corporation in 'Alien.' Completely fictional, of course. No company could possibly place profit over the lives of its people, right?

Nearly all of the heart transplant surgery was on April 7, which just happens to be the final day of the Battle of Shiloh in 1862, which my great-great grandpa barely survived. #secondbirthday

Eventually, he marched to the sea with General Sherman. Whenever I'm in Atlanta, I appreciate how good it looks after Nathaniel trashed it in 1864.

Julia: Which side was he on?

Me: Union. 12th Illinois Infantry. He was in the Hornets' Nest, the worst spot on the whole battlefield.

Maria: So, you are saying getting into some really shitty situations and surviving them is in your blood?

Alaena: Only on odd numbered years.

Maria: Well, no — if Battle of Shiloh was in 1862, and his great-great-grandfather survived, then even numbered years work, too.

Sarah: Beware the Ides of Odd!

Alaena: No, Terry only tries to die on odd-numbered years. Perhaps G-G-Grandpa was an even year-ed near-death kinda guy.

Maria: More research is clearly needed.

Virginia: My great-grandfather was there, too, and lived. He was on the losing side, my family being from east Tennessee. He had joined up at 16. After the war he went on to have 11 children. My grandfather, who passed when I was 12, was the 11th one born.

Not easy to twist your neck with a big-ass port in it. (photo 30)

Maria: WHERE is the lobster and the pink champagne? And, more importantly, the dancing girls?

The @#$! lobster drank the champagne and ran off with the dancing girls. Bastard.

Tina: WHO smuggled in the BelVita cookies? That's a TRUE friend (wife?)!

Janet: Since he has had only two meals since lunch on Saturday and it takes forever to get food, I figured these would work in a pinch.

Embracing the cannibal lifestyle was nearly a thing, but I figured getting Kuru disease wouldn't endear me to the Transplant Team.

Kuru is the human form of mad-cow disease, found in New Guinea cannibals from eating infected brains.

Up and moving with a Xmas tree full of lights. (photo 31)

Scott: And this is where those years of cycling and running pay off. Put a new motor in, and the rest of the machine is ready to ride. Bravo!

Cindi: I like that you're wearing a cape — Superman.

That's actually a second hospital gown, covering my bare, but spectacular, backside.

Mandy: You need a wizard hat to go with that robe....go careful please!

I had one. It assigned me to Hufflepuff.

Jim: They have you mowing the lawn already?

No, that's what they make the interns do.

We're moving again!

Off to the classier zip code of the ICU: Cardiac 90210.

(Janet) Not so fast. The nurse noticed a rash spot on his tummy and they have to consult infectious disease doctors before we move.

I do a lot of rash things.

Rebecca: Darn, reaction to a med?

Janet: Don't know. They have been arguing about something that popped up on the chart days ago and no one has made up their minds about it.

Melissa: A lot of people have a mild allergic reaction to adhesive tape from bandages.

Janet: It could be just adhesive tape with blood, it could a skin reaction to the tape, it could be a reaction to the shingles vaccine they gave him right before surgery. They won't decide till the doctor looks at it and we've been waiting for hours after packing up everything to move. And again, Terry gets no food.

(Janet) Infectious doctor said rash was nothing to worry about. Took some doing with all the hookups but we finally moved to room 371 in the ICU unit we started in, on the opposite side of the nurses' station. We can see the old room from the doorway. This is the swankier, but a bit less critical, section.

Back home at the main cardiac ICU again, only 49 hours after I left it. Well, not ALL of me came back.

Marisa: Were you able to keep your achy-breaky heart?

Christine: No way would they let him keep it. Amyloidosis is rare enough that there's probably a line of researchers out the door wanting a piece of it.

AE: Since it was so rare, hope you sold it for big bucks.

I wanted to auction it off to the Mayo Clinic, Sloan-Kettering, Beth Israel, and Massachusetts General, with sealed bids.

Maria: Oooh, could it have been a trade to pay for your hospital stay? A heart for a heart — very biblical.

Victoria: How are you feeling? Prayers for continued progress.

Me: Pretty much the same as when I was here the first time, only with nearly 10 drainage tubes in.

Cheri: Half the drainage but twice the fun?

4/10/19
(Janet) Terry is hurting this morning and having a hard time breathing. They have him on pain meds. It has only been Monday morning since he got out of surgery. They are calling him a rock star, but he is starting to get depressed. I'm going back to Alaena's house to ride out the storm due around noon. The change in pressure might be why Terry is hurting more.

I was marshaling my forces to annoy all of America with these FB posts again.

(Janet) I had been camped out on the couch in the rooms since Saturday and did not have a change of clothes, toothbrush, or hairbrush. I had to use the public bathroom down a long hallway ,which is very creepy to get to in the middle of the night. Reminded me of 'The Shining.'

Redrum!

Alaena: He doesn't deal with pressure change well, does he? This one is similar (though not quite) as bad as the last bomb cyclone.

Ali: There often seems to be a low point a day or two after any surgery. Probably a combination of heavy-duty meds wearing off, delayed shock, and return of sensation. Hopefully he'll be better tomorrow. Or, if still in serious pain, they may up the meds to get him mobile.

Julia: A friend told me the other evening, that depression often follows heart surgery. Don't worry much, it's normal. We're all cheering for him out here and appreciate the updates.

Ruth: When my father had open heart surgery (and therefore that same awful chest opening procedure) he had a lot of pain, and also became depressed for a time. It seems like that happens a lot. We hold a lot of emotion in our chests and it is such a huge and invasive procedure, that is really is no wonder that it affects him so deeply. Give him our love. It's a tough slog, but he's on the right side of the mountain now.

Karen: This too shall pass. Depression is normal. This just means the healing has begun. Terry, keep your chin up...it helps relieve the pressure...seriously. Use the meds and sleep as much as they will let you. Almost 4 years post and I still have pain, but it is the cost of doing business. You just have to find a way to occupy your mind. Might be time for a new hobby to go with that fabulous heart. Mine is jewelry making and coloring. Something that you have to use your hands and concentrate. It will make all the difference in your pain levels.

Just what I need, another hobby. I drive Janet nuts with the ones I already have/had: cycling, writing, curling, cricket, fencing, stage combat, Shakespearean acting, being fabulous...

Me: Feeling much better, now that 6 very uncomfortable items have been removed from my body. Sitting in a chair. Planning to walk later.

Nobody ever mentions the wretched drainage tubes that will take up 127% of your interior for a week after.

11 days in. (photo 32)

Grace: You look great! How long are they going to keep you?

Me: Until they're sure the heart is stable, not being rejected, and I have no other major health issues from the transplant.

Stable, not being rejected...sounds like a Taylor Swift song.

Jim: It's probably too late now, but this photo got me wondering about your donor's hair.

I'm more concerned about his aortic valve.

2 IV's, 3 drainage tubes, and the urinary catheter removed today. Doctors still beyond happy with the progress. 2 drainage tubes and pacemaker leads left to go. #quickhealer

Maria: Did they add more crap to your IV Christmas tree again?

Me: It constantly changes.

Maria: Ugh. I hope they are keeping a careful track.

Everything's labeled. Cord/tube management is 118% of a nurse's job. They must have recurrent nightmares about being dragged down to the depths by an IV-line kraken.

I may be making stellar progress, but my chest and arms look like props from *The Walking Dead*.

Julie: It's a good thing you have always been a character actor.

Curtis: How do you know they aren't?

No residual checks.

Just had my first hospital sponge bath, which was desperately needed. She removed the grunge but the various colors of medical soap stain on my right forearm were beyond anyone's powers.

In my ignorance, I didn't know what those really were. You'll notice that ignorance is a major theme here.

Me: I can see why people pay big money for spa pampering.

Me: Though your average spa worker probably doesn't discuss her 9 years in the Coast Guard while scrubbing your nether bits.

Maria: I SUPPOSE that qualifies as an emergency rescue of sorts.
Samantha: Coming from experience, nail polish remover gets tape residue off real well.

Marisa: But do not recommend in any open wounds.

They eventually sent me home with hospital-grade acetone wipes specifically made for that. I still have some left.

Well, the transplant jacked up my ejection fraction from 20% to 67%. FYI, that's about as good as EF (left ventricle pumping power) gets.

EF is how much blood the left ventricle pumps out to the rest of the body. For the average person, anything approaching 70% is great. It rarely gets above that, because there's always some left in the chamber after each contraction. Anything below 50-55% begins to be worrisome. Below 30% and alarm bells start going off.

Me: This heart beats so hard it rocks my head on the pillow.

♫ *"Rock me gently, rock me slowly…"*

Theresa: Teenagers. Don't know how good they have it. Hope his or her sacrifice gives you a fighting chance.

Maria: I am tired and misread this as "erection fraction"...which provoked a curious mental picture.

*Well, that, too, though I **was** going to leave it unmentioned. #notjoking*

Cheri: I'd need diagrams for this.

Didn't you get those in that awkward middle school health class?

Alaena: That's what I first read too. Uh, TMI!!!

Kathy: Ditto.

Linda: Same here.

Careful what you wish for, ladies. I'm on all sorts of crazy meds and can't be responsible for my actions.

Maria: You know...there is this proverb, "Tell me who your friends are, and I'll tell you who you are." Apparently, we all of us here are a bunch of perverted bastards. So, what does it tell us about Terry?

Me: Hey, don't blame me for a darned thing on this one.

I typed carefully and double-checked, for once.

Nancy: I did, too!!! I was all like, whoa! Who knew a new heart does that?!

Brian: 'Jacked up my ejection...' — yep, I thought that was kind of a weird, but good, by-product of the operation.

It's literally true, because the circulation goes from near-nothing to spectacular... everywhere.

Eileen: I've been in nursing too long. I saw it right the first time and missed all the fun. It's a hell of an EF, though. Enjoy that pulse, baby.

Hospitals are where dignity and self-respect go to die.

You know what really sucks after heart transplant surgery?

Hiccups. #ouch

Me: The nurse says it's distressingly common.

Debbie: Boo! (It used to work on the kids)

It'll take a lot more than that to scare me, after this experience.

Jill: After my C-section 27 years ago, my co-workers showed up with a stuffed gorilla. Towards the end of my pregnancy, I used to walk around the hospital singing the "Magilla Gorilla" song ("We've got a gorilla for sale...") because I actually lumbered when I walked. I'm a relatively small person and I was basically carrying around a watermelon in front of me. It was so hilarious I couldn't stop laughing, even though it hurt so much. And they kept laughing with me so it was this painful, but worthwhile, recursive loop.

"Laughter's the best medicine," my Aunt Fanny. (it doesn't help with diarrhea, either)

T: And sneezing.

Sneezing's worse. 50% more pressure on the sternum than coughing.

Hope: Eat a spoonful of sugar. Seriously. It worked like magic. I had hiccups after surgery (not nearly as extensive surgery, to be fair) but it still hurt like hell.

It seriously concerns me that we're taking our medical advice from Mary Poppins now. Could be worse, could be Nanny McPhee.

4/11/19
The movie playing on the hospital TV as I was wheeled off for my heart transplant was *Iron Man*. Oddly apropos. Well, except for the billionaire part. And the mechanical heart part. And the cool dude part. And...

Kelly: You're awake early.

Me: Nobody sleeps in a hospital, especially me, since I have a port in my neck connected to an IV and can't turn over.

Maria: Listen, Tony Stark was never cool enough to rock an Elizabethan ruff collar. It takes you!

Remember, it's the bejeweled codpiece that maketh the man.

Janet: I can attest to the not sleeping in the hospital part, having stayed in the rooms from Saturday to Wednesday. Every two hours, at least, someone comes in. Though I slept at Alaena's last night, and the supersized snow ploughs, with flashing colored lights scraping ice and snow up and down the hill about 6 to 8 times, spooked the dog so much at 4 a.m. that it took hugging time on the couch before she went back to sleep.

"Mama! The noisy flashy monster-thingy's a-comin' to get me! Only doggy bacon can fight it!"

Well, yes, I suppose getting a heart transplant WAS a long way to go to get out of proctoring the SAT test yesterday.

Russell: Worth it, I'd say.

Sarah: I'd rather have a transplant!

Apparently, this hospital's portable X-ray machines only function between 1 and 5 a.m. Must be a factory defect.

Rebecca: I worked 11 to 7 for years. We hate doing them too, when you get 15 orders for 5 a.m. you have to start early. It is so everything is ready for the doctor.

Yeah, yeah, yeah, all for the doctor. Like they're saving lives or something.

Smoochies! My heart beats only for you, honeybunch.

No joke to be made here.

4 wires from the temporary external pacemaker yanked out of my chest just now, along with an IV in the artery of my wrist. Tomorrow the big external electric pump and attending hose comes out of the incision area (it encourages healing somehow). Today I should also get most of the extra neck port junk removed, though the port itself and the last drainage tube have to stay in until the heart biopsy on Monday. Might get off of the last IV line today and be off leash, just on oral meds ('just': it's a mind-boggling assortment). Doctors are all happy at the data they're seeing so far. Considering how many ways there are for this transplant business to go horribly wrong, that's what I want to hear.

Off to do laps in the hall in my sexy yellow hospital socks.

Somehow no one threw themselves at me in erotic abandon at the sight of those socks. Weird.

Me: That said, there are still 7 bags hanging on my IV pole.

Jay: Great news. Lots of progress. Lots of other colors of socks to have chosen from but yellow is for caution. Be careful.

Bill: Great news. Just keep those 19-year-old urges in check for a while.

Believe me, if hospitals slay dignity, they slay romance even more.

Maria: Yeah, Terry, this is one time we don't want you to be strange or original. No exceptions. No surprises. By the book. Off you go.

Kate: Wait, what? A heart biopsy? They're going to go in after a little piece of your new heart? Sheesh! They already got the old one to play with.

It's a sort of cardiology tax, I think. A literal excise tax, in fact.

Jim: Do tell — about those sexy yellow hospital socks...are they cross-gartered?

An allusion to the absurd Malvolio in Shakespeare's 'Twelfth Night.'

Me: I'll have to order that little detail from Malvolio's Cut-Rate Hospital Supply.

Judith: In the olden days when my dad had a triple bypass, he was bed-ridden for three full weeks — look how far we have come since the 80's.

John: Did you take that one last chance to jack into the Matrix before they pulled your neck port?

*I'm pretty sure they make me take the red **and** the blue pills. In fact, Mycophenelate (anti-rejection) has both colors on one capsule (okay, blue and orange...close enough).*

My fancy-schmancy hospital bong. (photo 33)

Stephanie: I have one just like it! Maybe we should have a contest. Or not.

John: Keep going — you'll be a Mercury astronaut before you know it.

An allusion to Scott Glenn as Alan Shepard in the movie 'The Right Stuff.' The astronauts had to blow into a water-filled tube and keep a ping-pong ball hovering as long as they could. When they all eventually gave up, Shepard was still casually, um, blowing them out of the water.

Victoria: For four million dollars, it better be.

Alas, I get nothing but an oxygen high from it. Oh, and a lack of pneumonia.

All IV lines removed. I'm off the leash. They may let me walk around unescorted tomorrow.

Or maybe not. The 2 laps I just did were a wretched slog. The body hasn't gotten over the outrage yet. Only been 4 days.

Debbie: Wow, you make it sound so easy. Drove up to a transplant window, picked up a heart to go. Done...........Next!

I do want fries with it. Thanks for asking. And do you have any of those little Prednisone packets?

Maria: WHOA! No yellow sock racing now. Behave!

Marisa: No longer a cyborg?

Literally the first time in 2 years that some sort of electronic medical device hasn't been keeping me going.

AE: Wow! I am amazed! Are you sure you are following doctors' orders and not just unleashing yourself when no one is looking??? Hmm...

The only place to walk is around the ICU main desk. Pretty sure they'd notice if I was being unruly.

4/12/19
If doesn't inspire confidence that the nurse had to put on a hazmat suit to plug in one of my IV meds this morning.

Julie: Was it for your protection or hers?

Sessha: They do the same thing at chemo. It is because they are exposed so often to so many different meds.

Barbara: I never saw hazmat suits used at my hospital. We just use the yellow gowns and gloves.

Me: That's what I'm calling that getup.

I notice that nobody offered me that protection. In fact, they injected all manner of horrifying stuff straight into my veins like it was an illicit Nazi experiment.

I'm on TWENTY different medications right now.

"Mycophenolate mofetil: it's part of a balanced breakfast."

Tim: I left the hospital on 16 different meds. I'm down to 13 now.

Me: Some of these are post-op hospital use and will go away.

As of now I have about 12 different meds, I think. 3 for rejection; the rest are for the side-effects of those or of the transplant itself: for unclogging arteries, hypertension, pneumonia, CMV virus, thrush infection, osteoporosis, depression, hypothyroidism, and abdominal distress. A handful every 12 hours. Some are a.m., some p.m., some both. Some will taper off and be gone soon.

"We have figured out how to rip the beating heart out of someone and cram it into another person's chest. Why don't we have a cure for hiccups yet?" (FB meme)

Apparently, the medical community is unaware of Mary Poppins' cutting-edge research in this arena.

Just did 5 laps around the cardiac ICU, all at once, nothing holding me up. That's my all-day expectation from Physical Therapy. I told the doctors and nurses I was doing a walkathon and they all owed me $.

Gretchen: Hang in there, my friend. You have a world of people, lots of theatre geeks, Shakespeare enthusiasts, and students sending you vibes, prayers, and good juju.

Adorable. (Photo 34)

Rebecca: I assume that is your cough pillow.

Me: They ran out of their official heart pillows, so I'm using a tightly rolled up towel. This is a toy sent to me, Harry the Heart.

Rebecca: Harry is very cute.

Mark: Looks like the Face Hugger missed. Good to see you without all the tubes running into your head.

Joshwa: Glad you're recovering...but shouldn't they put your heart inside of your chest?

You clearly haven't stayed abreast of the newest research in the field. We're using voodoo now.

Cindi: I had a dentist appointment today. I have a phobia about dentists. But today I told myself, if Terry Kroenung can go through a heart transplant, 1 can suffer through the dentist without freaking out. It helped.

♬ "Son, you'll be a dentist, you have a talent for causing things pain. You'll be a dentist, people will pay you to be inhumane..."

Yes, 1 worked in a bit of 'Little Shop of Horrors', a perfect name for this place.

Face washed, hair brushed (sort of), shaved, teeth brushed & flossed.

Control yourselves, ladies. (photo 35)

Me: It's the jugular vein port, right? Chicks dig that.

Lincoln: Chicks dig the long tube.

You have no idea. When they pulled it out, I thought the other end was down in my left foot.

Julie: Uh, you're married, but you're kinda cute.

More kinda than cute.

"A little more than kin and less than kinda." – 'Hamlet', the revised hospital edition.

Garalt: He's got the pump of a 19-year-old, alright.

Ali: When they take it out, you'll need to get a bolt to keep up the image.

A fine suggestion, as it turned out. A bolt from the blue.

Julie: Ooowweee, damn Terry, that mustache and beard are HOT! Does your wife need backup to fight off the nurses and aides?

Me: Not so far. Nothing less alluring than having watch an old guy pee several times a day and then record the amount he produces.

Julie: Be still my heart. Wait....

Scott: Is that a jugular port in your neck or are you just happy to see me?

It's called a Swan, short for Swan-Ganz catheter. It's in the jugular vein and snakes through the right ventricle, right atrium, and into the pulmonary artery.

Then I think it goes through the wall at Platform 9 3/4 and into Hogwarts.

Perry: That 19-year-old heart is gonna pump blood into places that will get you into trouble if you're not careful.

Sharon: Ooo-la-la…but I prefer the legs and Big Bird feet!

I was kind of hoping for Oscar the Grouch socks. A better fit for me.

The tech game is strong with the vampires of Anschutz Med Center.

I get great TV reception on it. (photo 36)

Kelly: What's that do?

Me: They put meds into it, take blood out without needling me again, and will do the Monday biopsy through it.

Kelly: What're they looking for with the biopsy?

Jimmy Hoffa, I think.

Christine: Any early signs of rejection.

Alaena: He will be getting biopsies at decreasing intervals for life. Once a week starting next week.

Kelly: Wow!

Garalt: Low budget Locutus. Probably cost more than the entire third season of *Star Trek:TNG*.

The first season, anyway, from what I hear.

Mandy: Ow.

Me: Doesn't hurt at all. They put it in when I was totally out.

Along with both urinary catheters. Totally lucked out on all of that.

As a teacher of 30 years, I've learned to always keep a supply of staples on hand. (photo 37)

Me: That's where they took out the pacemaker.

Rebecca: Wait till you see the chest. Imagine the stories you can tell about all the scars.

Me: "You should see the other guy."

Cheri: I prefer to keep my staples in the supply closet, but this also works.

Maria: OWWWWWW! That one just looks like Dracula had had his way with you.

Barbara: And I bet they hurt with the slightest move.

Me: Not really.

Bill: I take it they removed your port. Too bad. I've always wanted a built-in USB port.

This was more the size of the Port Authority Bus Terminal.

Me: The neck monstrosity is still there.

Janet: The lower arm bruises are quite the sight too.

Alaena: You should get pictures of your wrists. That's some serious Technicolor there.

So, you know how fun peeling a tenacious band-aid is? Imagine the unadulterated joy of having your heart transplant dressing stripped off? Slowly.
#thatgotmyattention #couldhavebeenworse

It was basically medical duct tape.

Marti: At least you won't have to wax your chest this week!

Or possibly ever again.

Julie: How high did your eyebrows go?

Karen: I can't breathe just thinking about it.

Maria: There ought to be a separate set of anesthetics for this.

Hey, boss, I need some time off. Here's my doctor's note. (photo 38)

Me: You know the scene in *Jaws* where they compare scars? I win.

Veronica: I don't know. I've got a scar from a flip flop.

Dean: Those escaping xenomorphs really make a mess, don't they?

Kathryn: That's so punk rock, Terry!

Me: More like *Hellraiser.*

Kathryn: "We have all eternity to zip your chest..."

Patti: Are those staples?

Me: Looks like a mix of staples and sutures.

Turned out to be only staples. 50 of them.

Julie: Is that a zipper ?!

Ah, another epiphany provided by my FB friends.

David: Duct tape. And get back to work.

Cerene: Malikai got a kick out of your battle scars. Had to explain the use of the heart-lung machine as to why you didn't die when they took out the old heart.

Debbie: Well, your boobs are even....good plastic surgery job!!!

Russell: Please bear in mind that in the U.K. it's breakfast time. Right off my muesli, now.

Don't try that with me. You guys eat blood pudding and fry up kidneys.

Michael: You could have a very convincing Frankenstein costume this Halloween.

Pat: I wonder if heart surgeons think about that scene in *The Thing* when they go in.

The scene is question has a doctor working on a patient's chest, but said patient is actually a shape-shifted alien. An enormous shark-toothed mouth opens up and chomps off both his arms. One of my favorite comedic moments from this uproarious gem.

Mark: You should put a zipper tattoo on the top of your incision. Would make a great conversation piece.

Me: I can have Janet paint that on. No tattoos when you're immune-suppressed.

David: Zippers are so last century! Maybe a nice Velcro enclosure?

Mark: "'Tis but a scratch..."

Me: "I've had worse."

More Monty Python. Witty banter from the King Arthur/Black Knight duel. The knight has lost an arm.

Garalt: No xenomorph, no day off. We need physical evidence.

I have a bulb full of blood draining out of me. Is that good enough?

4/13/19
One of the little joys of extensive hospital IV use: that's not dirt, that's a bruise.

Weirdly, no bruising where they opened me up with a car jack. (photo 39)

This is actually one of those instances where leeches made sense.

Julia: Ouch. Look at it this way - the blood is pumping there.

Me: Yeah, and a lot harder and faster than before.

Donna: I know, eh? I was thinking how good your colour was looking post-op!

Liana: That'll take a while to reabsorb.

Weeks and weeks, ultimately. The vein still hasn't recovered.

Julie: You are not allowed to bruise! Stop it immediately! (mom-eyes)

It's part of my secret identity. I'm Bruise Wayne.

Alaena: Kinda pretty in a twisted sort of way.

AE: Colorful — soon you will be a rainbow.

Victoria: Thank you. My special effects students have been practicing and I think you're pretty close.

Glad to be of service, ma'am.

Kudos to writer Cindy Myers for knowing intuitively what I needed. Clearly, she was paying attention when we were on those author panels. The doctors all think it's a hoot. (photo 40)

Courtney: Uh ... I want one of these.

Me: Amazon, $7.59. It's just a low-rent puzzle book with profane instructions. Don't expect much beyond the cover. That's all Cindy knew about it.

This title would be used for 'The Great Gatsby' and make perfect sense.

So, this just happened. The head cardiologist came in and said when they inspected the old heart (which was spectacularly awful and DID

have to come out, **BTW**), it didn't look like a typical heart with amyloidosis. It looked like there was also sarcoidosis, an infiltrative auto-immune thing. So they sent chunks off to the Mayo Clinic for analysis.

He also said that I'm the only patient **EVER** to require 3 nuclear imaging scans to get a diagnosis, even though it was wrong. That's me, a living medical school test case.

Barbara: I know you can get sarcoidosis in the lungs, but I didn't know about the heart.

Me: Lungs are clear as a bell. Healthiest thing about me, they say.

Alaena: Hopefully they tell you what they find. Will be interested to find out.

Me: My best bet is a subtle alien invasion.

Li: I've known several people have sarcoidosis affect their lungs. For some reason, everything seems to have headed for your heart. Wonder which you got first. One of the theories about auto-immune and inflammatory diseases is that they may be an adaptation of extra vigilant immune system that helped children survive crowded polluted conditions in the past few hundred years. And although these 'modern' diseases tend to affect middle class people, it often turns out their ancestors a few generations back were not in such good conditions.

Melisse: I have pulmonary sarcoidosis, but it is in remission. However, I do have diminished lung capacity. Am following an anti-inflammatory diet.

Cerene: Always knew you were an oddball at heart.

Me: Pot/kettle, dear.

Cerene: TAKES ONE TO KNOW ONE.

Maria: You sound like a living, breathing episode of *House MD*.

Not sure that's a good thing. He had an opioid addiction. I hope my doctors aren't also over-sampling their product.

Dave: Sarcoidosis along with amyloidosis. There's a hell of a duo.

Me: I don't dick around.

Veronica: Sooooooo...we need to ask for your autograph next time we see you?

I only sign bosoms and butts. Sorry, it's a hospital rule.

Told the wife the other day that since the heart transplant, she's technically in a manage á trois. The eye roll caused a tsunami on the Japanese coast.

I'm told there are photos of my old, diseased heart. Stay tuned.

Me: Adjust your mealtime Facebook viewing accordingly.

Ali: Seriously, I remember years ago they broadcast open-heart surgery on breakfast TV.

Eileen: I'm a trauma nurse. That IS mealtime viewing.

I used to thumb through forensic medicine textbooks at the dinner table. My popularity was somehow not enhanced.

Alaena: Oddly looking forward to that.

Ali: Yuck. Thinking of various songs involving heart you could use to make a bad video.

Julie: Eewwwww! Ewww, eeeww, ewwwwwww! Let me see.

Cal: Book. You have a big audience already. Heart disease is still the #1 killer for both men and women. And you survived to tell the story.

The heart transplant was 6 days ago.
I just walked a mile...unaccompanied.

Update: And another 1/2-mile before dinner. #fearme

Cheri: Are you sure you're not actually a cyborg?

Positive. I have the removal incision to prove it. Granted, I didn't actually see what they sewed into me. Maybe it's a lawnmower engine.

Julie: That is astounding! Just don't overdo it, as you are prone to do.

Me: It's not overdoing it until I'm actually prone.

David: You walked a mile? That's great. But how did you get back to the hospital?

Me: Uber.

Lincoln: Dude! If you keep this up, Nike will be offering you a gazillion dollar endorsement deal!

Don't you have to be really fast, or take a knee, or something?

Just watched the scene in *Last of the Mohicans* where the British colonel gets his beating heart cut out by the vengeful Indian warlord. What's up with this hospital's programming choices in my transplant week?

Janet: I bet they didn't show that *Star Trek* Picard episode.

He took a Klingon knife to the chest. Had to get a mechanical one put in (a heart, not a knife).

Me: It'll be an Aztec documentary on the History Channel next.

Eileen: "Sponsored by the anesthesiology department."

Cardio-Thoracic Surgery department, more likely. A bunch of zany wags over there .

Me: *Merchant of Venice* will be next.

Scott: *Six Million Dollar Man?*

Jenn: *Indiana Jones and The Temple of Doom?*

Shannon: *Dances with Wolves.*

Maria: Is that like a warning to you — in case you don't behave?

(Meme) "I feel like I'm in season 5 of my life and the writers are just making ridiculous shit happen to keep it interesting."

Me: My students have always accused me of doing crazy shit just to be more interesting than they are. Pretty sure I can't top this, short of an alien abduction live on CNN.

I seem to be fixated on alien abductions in this book. Must be my, um, probing intellect.

(The perfect meme for what these exotic meds are doing to me) "You ever see the movie *Constipation*? No? That's because it hasn't come out yet." Between the surgical trauma and the exotic medicinal cocktail, my poor bowels moved like molasses in Antarctica.

It took a week to even begin to clear out, despite the state-of-the-art IV laxatives and pills they kept dumping into me. Everybody kept asking me about it daily with great earnestness. Maybe they thought I was going to poop diamonds.

4/14/19
That's right, I just went mano a mano with the suck machine (manual incentive spirometer) and kicked its ass. Maxed it out at 4000. #lungsofsteel

Me: Proof that hospital living literally sucks.

Liana: Sometimes it blows!

My cardiac resident is rotating out tomorrow. I gave her minor misery for being named Knees and not being an orthopedist. She won the duel by rubbing it in that she was going to Iceland and Dublin and I...wasn't.

Tina: Ding*ding*ding*   —   Resident   wins,   hands   down!

If all goes well with the heart biopsy tomorrow (checking for signs of rejection), I may be home Tuesday.

Rebecca: Could you post your home address, so it won't get lost in the hospital?

Me: I can only lift 10 pounds. I'm not up to lugging enormous stacks of fan mail yet.

Alaena: While I still think they are pushing your release a smidge, your Uber has cleared her schedule for Tuesday. Keep me updated so I may have your carriage ready.

Hopefully it's not an enchanted pumpkin pulled by transmogrified mice. Because I don't have glass slippers, just these goofy yellow socks.

Janet: I think they are pushing it, too. From experience, hospital discharge is a lengthy, complicated process, so a specific time on Tuesday may be hard to determine.

Scott: Agreed. One thing I learned from major infrastructure projects — saying the start date is easy, projecting the completion date is hard and frequently perilous.

Suzann: They told a very impatient Ken that he was going home by noon and at 4:30 pm we were still there waiting for everyone to sign off. He was so upset.

Janet: We had that problem when he had the pacemaker put in and when he had the PICC line put in. He was so upset he threatened to pull out the tubes and just leave. He was supposed to leave in the morning and they had him hooked up to tubes at 7 p.m. that night.

That let them charge for the room an extra day, I'm guessing.

Unless you're very local (and possibly not even then), you probably shouldn't send anything to me at the hospital now, as it looks like I'll be discharged Tuesday. Instead, send it to my palatial manor, where we've laid on extra servants to handle the volume.

Rebecca: Give everybody else the right address this time.

Me: It's the 20 different meds, I swear.

Rebecca: I knew you would blame it on that. Your neighbors may be getting a package.

Maria: Hey, do you have any dietary restrictions?

No fried placentas.

Me: Minimal. Grapefruit is gone forever, it screws up the immunosuppression.

Me: We have a basset hound. NO food will be wasted.

Maria: Can the basset hound have grapefruit?

Janet: Abby will not eat anything resembling fruit. Won't eat corn chips either.

Janet: Oh, and I read that pomegranate is restricted, also.

Janet: Your one servant now has to alert the mail person and the neighbor that you screwed up the address.

Hey, maybe I noticed the neighbor was sad and lonely and could use some loving mail. Ever think of that?

The charge nurse just came in and said they have Sock ID here. All the time I've been wearing the tres fashionable bright yellow socks, that was code for the staff for 'high fall risk' and somebody should've been dragging me back to bed, despite being cleared to walk on my own. I'm now been promoted to the brown 'do whatever the hell you want, we're too understaffed to stare at your damned feet' socks.

Sock ID. It's like Caller ID, only not as fantastically on trend.

Sharon: I was given yellow Big Bird feet when I had neck surgery. High fall risk…true.

Beth: You need to frame those socks!!

I did. Their attempted murder trial starts next week.

Pamela: I never knew that the colors meant anything! What's blue mean?

Me: It likely varies with the hospital. Probably intermediate fall risk here.

Maria: Yup, varies by hospital. But bright, easily noticeable colors — red, yellow, and orange — are usually for something important as in "come grab this person RIGHT NOW!" Also, at our hospital, nurses distributing medication wear a yellow ribbon over their shoulder — it means "please don't distract this person, she is delivering meds, we don't want your Valium to go to someone else, do we?" It seriously reduced the number of medication errors. There are usually signs posted around hospitals using this type of color coding — telling people what to do if, for instance, they see a person in orange socks walking unattended. They should stop the person, send someone to get a nurse, and stay with that person until the nurse comes.

Yellow ribbon: Good system. Mixing up the morphine with the suppository would be…unfortunate.

Multiple nurses kept offering me suppositories for the drug-fueled constipation. I can only guess that there was a substantial financial bonus for administering them.
Bill: I can't wait till you graduate back to your own argyle socks.

I have numerous pairs of those, actually, mostly for Steampunk cosplay. Have to wear them sparingly, as I can't be responsible for their amatory effect.

Victoria: The funny thing is, those are great socks. Whenever I've had surgery, I bring them home and wear them around the house. No slipping on my floors and they keep my feet nice and toasty in the cold without getting too hot. Take home as many as you can — they are great! Interesting about the color coding.

Not a fan of them for extended use on tile floors. The rubbery non-slip nubs on the bottom dig into my feet. Plus, the elastic isn't great and they tend to work themselves down and bunch up under my foot (which at least pads those nasty nubs).

Cal: You remind me of Snoopy's creator Charles Schulz — a lovely man who I interviewed a few times. He had heart surgery and used his sense of humor during his stay. The cartoonist even drew Snoopy on the wall, per a nurse's request.

Me: I had a Disney artist draw the Lion King on my classroom whiteboard.

Maria: I think brown stands for "you are full of it — you are going to go out on your own anyhow, so we just give up!"

Rebecca: I think blue is the default color of all hospitals. I have never heard of the sock/fall system, but it does not seem to work.

Mark: At the hospital I work at, we have bright orange bracelets that indicate a fall risk. The color of sock (gray, tan, blue, orange, and green) just indicates what size foot you have.

Erin: I'm actually surprised that you weren't wearing compression socks so as to prevent DVT.

Deep vein thrombosis. Blood clots in the lower legs from not moving much.

Me: They did that earlier.

Erin: Fair enough. Then I'm surprised that you have them off so quickly. Here you basically wear them for weeks afterwards. And I think would be recommended to wear them for the rest of your life, as it were.

They don't seem concerned about that at all. Maybe because I'm much more likely to fall victim to a cycling accident, sword mishap, or being suffocated by an Eeyore plushie avalanche.

Julie: Now I want to get my family new socks and have a secret color code they only discover in my will.

"And to my loving brother in the magenta stockings, I leave all my Tupperware. Guard it tenaciously."

Joe: I was on the same protocol in UC Loveland Hospital last summer for 10 of the 12 days I was there. I didn't even know about it till the 11th day! LOL

This is Day 15 for me.

New day nurse just came in with a mask on and announced that she was going home, as she was sicker than I was. Told her I might go home on the 8th day post-transplant. Her response was, "That's insane."

I wasn't sure if she meant the discharge or just me in general.

Janet: I think it's a bit optimistic, too.

Rebecca: I do not envy you for the next few weeks trying to keep him busy.

Julia: How about keeping him down?

Me: You can't keep me down. I have the BROWN socks!!!

Marisa: Geez, aren't you supposed to avoid sick people? Like no sick nurses near the patients with compromised immune systems!

Me: Well, that's one way to look at it.

Just walked a pre-breakfast mile in 24 minutes, 8 or 9 minutes quicker than yesterday. Average 96 bpm on the ticker.

Alaena: Your new ticker and your brain have not learned to work together yet. Said bragging is meaningless.

Me: The doctors and nurses are all fine with it, so...pfftth!

Barbara: I'm guessing you didn't have any shortness of breath, and if I'm right that was awesome.

Me: Nope.

Sarah: Careful, they're going to give you the lead socks just to slow you down.

They'll have to 'Harrison Bergeron me' to stop me.

"Harrison Bergeron" is a 1961 science-fiction short story by Kurt Vonnegut, where everyone, by law, must be completely equal in every way. Those with great talent or skill or intellect have government-installed handicap so they won't have an advantage. The title character is so gifted, and a rebel to boot, that he is burdened by 300 lbs. of equality weights.

Jim: Are they preparing you to walk home?

Me: Might as well, there's NO parking here.

The throbbing nerve center of the Cardiac ICU, mission control for Heart Central, the vital engine that keeps...um. Hope no emergency happens. What's the likelihood, though? (photo 41)

Janet: Busy in all the rooms taking care of patients?

Me: Oh, sure, take **their** side.

Might be getting an 'actual real water & shampoo, not just an alcohol wipe down shower' today. Haven't had that since around March 29.

Scott: A "Hollywood shower," huh? (Yes, my dad is former submarine service.) More progress!

I hope 'Hollywood shower' doesn't mean I get knifed by a cross-dressing Norman Bates. Because I've been knifed enough this week.

More like a cable-access TV shower, having seen the thing.

Debbie: Yeah...I was going to talk to you about that.

I don't doubt that the unfortunate odor reaches you in Canada.

My daily cardio team, in here every morning, 7 days a week. Dr. Knees on the left, Dr. Ambardekar, the amyloidosis expert and transplant boss, on the right. Sorry, middle guy, I've never known who you are. (photo 42)

AE: Poor middle guy. We know you as the "transplant doc in room 371 — that guy"

Me: If aliens attack the hospital , he's the redshirt.

Mark: Where's Dr. Gumby?

Me: Not here yet. He's too...pokey.

Mark: No...the Monty Python Dr. Gumby. Too many drugs, my friend.

Can there be too many drugs, really?

*On discharge day I was thoroughly disabused of **that** notion.*

Linda: What is amyloidosis?

Me: Liver makes too much transthyretin protein, clogs and destroys the heart.

Linda: So it was your old heart doing that?

Me: Yep, the ungrateful little bastard. So into the dustbin it went. Not all of it. Some went to the Mayo Clinic, since it's rare, especially mine.

Jim: Seal it with a baboon's blood, then the charm is firm and good!

Leave it to my stage combat partner of 20 years to drop the 'Macbeth' reference like a mic at a rap battle.

I'm a little bit pouty that we don't get therapy dogs up here. I want 3 drooling basset hounds slinging healing drool in all directions.

Maria: The extra drool could be used as free moisturizer!

Or mucilage.

AE: Which is why they don't let those guys in! Topper's fav thing to do when I'm in bed is sit on my chest — probably not wise in your case.

Bassets like to stand on your chest with their ears and jowls pendulously hanging in your face so you can't breathe. It's the only time they can look down on anything.

Stuck in a chair for 2 hours with a tube pouring spectacularly expensive goo into my neck. You know, a normal Sunday here.

Linda: ♫ "Living the glamorous life!"

A lyric from Stephen Sondheim's 'A Little Night Music,' based on a Swedish sex farce, of course.

Me: I'm free! Free!

But not easy.

Ali: In a Roger Daltrey way, or John Inman?

Jim: They are draining your essence for the king.

Too late. Elvis has left the building.

"A foreign substance is introduced into our precious bodily fluids without the knowledge of the individual, and certainly without any choice. That's the way your hard-core Commie works." – General Jack D. Ripper, 'Dr. Strangelove.'

This makes me happy. Number of years my heart is younger than the rest of me: 42. My heart is the answer to Life, the Universe, and Everything (at least for me; your mileage may vary). Just did another 1-mile walk, and had a nap.

Eileen: Your knees are gonna be jealous as hell.

Brian: Douglas Adams would be pleased.

Me: Ironically, he passed away from a sudden heart attack.

Maria: Don't forget your towel.

Well, that solid week of heroic intervention by the International Physicians' Laxative Brigade is finally paying off.

Tina: We love you, but we can pass on any pics — ahahahahahahaha!

Don't fear science, Tina. It's your friend.

Janet: They have been very interested in the BMs, haven't they?

Me: Five — FIVE — episodes Sunday. I lost half my body weight.

Dave: So you made Trump's new cabinet...okay...

Me: No, my commode production is still massively over-qualified.

Harriet: Well, we knew you were sometimes full of it, but this is crazy!!

The irony is that my fantasy novels always contain monsters made of magically-animated poop.

The Health Nazis cancelled my shower until after the biopsy tomorrow morning. Some trivial foolishness about possible infection and a miserable dreary death.

Julia: We still love you, shower or not.

*Sure, you say that **now**…*

Ana: What about the tube in your neck? Would they let you in the shower with that?

Me: That's the issue.

Ali: Guess you'll have to be dry-cleaned again.

Me: I've noticed that it went from a slow honeymoon experience to them tossing the packs of wipes at me and saying, "Here. Knock yourself out."

David: Sponge bath!

You say that with the sort of glee that leads me to make sure security doesn't admit you.

Precisely 7 days ago, about to the minute, I was on a gurney being wheeled into pre-op to have an ugly, festering growth removed from my manly (ish) chest so they could drop in a shiny new model.

10 minutes ago I finished walking my 3rd mile of the day. #itain'tyourgrandpa'smedicine

Eric: So Terry, because you've stayed in shape, is it that you didn't have any cardiovascular problems in your arteries, etc. besides the heart itself? Also, if you're already walking 3 miles, it sounds like they must've given you the Energizer Bunny heart.

Well, I do have a cute pink butt. Just sayin'…

Me: The crazy conditioning is helping now, but it also masked the severity of the illness until almost too late.

4/15/19
Not that it ever entered my mind, but I'm not allowed to fully-embrace the Colorado lifestyle now. Marijuana interferes with the uptake of anti-rejection meds. #runner'shighitisthen

Maria: Well, there goes your social life!

Me: Like I had one before.

Terry W.: That's interesting. Who knew?

Me: Who the hell did the research?

Doctor (firing up a fattie): "Relax, it's for science. Now, first question: Does this make your joints hurt?" Transplant patient: "Only if I put the burning end in my mouth."

Johnnie: Have they mentioned beer?

Mark: Ask about shrooms.

Remember, you can't spell 'fungus' without f-u-n.

Into Week 3 of my residency at this ultra-exclusive resort, apparently run by Shylock.

"Welcome to our hotel restaurant. If it feed nothing else, it will feed my revenge."

Speaking of Shylock, it occurs to me that I have to edit a story for the next Rocky Mountain Fiction Writers anthology, since submissions will be due soon. I kid you not, it's a Steampunk version of *The Merchant of Venice*, with Shylock being a vengeful automaton living in an airship above a ruined Earth post-HG Wells Martian invasion. Weird timing on that one.

Duly entered by the deadline. Still waiting for a yes or no.

Erin: I thought you wrote that one like 8 or 9 years ago? I seriously remember you having written that when I first became FB friends.

Me: They keep accepting it, but then they take one of my other stories instead to be fair to other authors who don't get 2 in one anthology. #embarrassment of riches

Ali: How much does a heart weigh?

Me: Just over 1/2 pound.

*My old one was **way** beyond that, alas.*

Ali: Plenty of scope for a pound of flesh, then.

After being assaulted by military-grade IV diuretics for the past week, all of my post-op edema is gone and I'm back to my usual scrawny less-than-160-lbs self. I'd been so swollen my shoes would never have fit. #noglassslipper

Edema: swelling from fluid accumulating in the tissues. Heart failure can cause it, but in my case, it was the surgery itself. Makes you look like the Sta-Puft Marshmallow man.

So if the transplant surgery had gone horribly wrong, my last words would've been "Look at this fancy-ass NASA setup!" #wordstoliveby

Mark: So long as they had the machine that goes 'Ping!'

Me: Every freaking machine here goes ping, non-stop.

Veronica: So beautiful. *wipes tear*

Janet: Not just ping. Every machine has its own alarm sound.

Nothing like having catheters run up into your beating heart to gouge out tissue samples to give you the full glorious experience of Tax Day. #nowthat'sametaphor

Jim: Since most of us aren't in a position for that experience, a colonoscopy would be an acceptable option.

It took a lotta guts to post that.

Victoria: You won the Internet today!

Veronica: Give unto Caesar, dude...

Don't want Caesar clawing at my myocardium. I'm particular that way.

Ali: Yuck. At least they'd already made the hole in your neck.

Mark: Hey, if ya gotta be probed, could be worse.

If the aliens hadn't sworn me to silence, I could tell you stories…

Looks like my current post-transplant med plan is at least 24 pills a day, plus some that aren't taken daily.

And as I type this, 12 ½ weeks out, they've switched a bunch of them again. My doctors should play 3-card monte.

Me: I'll rattle when I walk.

Maria: I know the anti-rejection stuff is for life, but are any of the other ones going away eventually?

Me: Some. A lot are to counteract the effects of the rejection meds.

Christine: "You take the blue pill, the story ends. You take the red pill, you stay in Wonderland, and I show you how deep the rabbit-hole goes."

Still waiting to magically acquire my kung fu and bullet-dodging skills.

After the biopsy today, I will have had about 20 hours of surgical procedures done since arriving at Chez Anschutz.

They do know how to show a fellow a good time. It's up to 24 hours now.

When they started my heart biopsy they were playing 'The Cell Block

Tango' from *Chicago* ("He ran into my knife...ten times"). When I woke up Mary Magdalene was singing to Jesus from *Jesus Christ Superstar* while I stared into a bright light.

"Welcome to the afterlife. You had some...complications."

Janet: And while you were out, Notre Dame in Paris caught fire.

Me: I have an alibi.

Biopsy all done, absurd ports removed from my neck. Now I just look like I'm in thrall to the Colorado Vampire Coven.

Stephany: It is mind-boggling what you have been through in the past two months. I am so glad that they identified the problem and fixed it, so we get to keep you around for a long time to come.

Janet: If it weren't for the doctor who runs the transplant center, I don't know if they would have figured it out right away. He came back from a heart conference in Florida, looked at the tests and said, 'New heart!' last Thursday. Lo and behold, a new heart on Sunday night. The doctors from the cardiology department in Loveland, who put in the pacemaker, are all calling me since I called in this morning to ask about what to do with the pacemaker equipment. They seem fascinated.

Andrew: Must be a relief every time they take another piece of equipment out of your body. I've only ever had a drain in my neck and when they took that out it hurt like hell. Can hardly imagine what it's all been like.

9 drains in your torso are a treat, let me tell you. I looked like the Flying Spaghetti Monster. #heboiledforyour sins

Christine: I'm curious, without the neck port, how will future biopsies be done?

Me: Like the diagnostic catheterization I had when this all started. Numb the neck, run the catheter in without all of that semi-permanent structure.

The pre-op prep is 3 times as long as the actual biopsy, which is all of 5 minutes. The *nurses do all of the work. The MD flies in to do his/her bit, gets paid $1200, then he/she glides on out for a latte.*

Alaena: That is until the veins in his neck are inaccessible due to scar tissue. Then they switch to the groin. He gets a crap ton of biopsies the first year and then a minimum once a year until the 19- year-old heart quits ticking.

Gary: If you were a computer, they would sell you as rebuilt.

Me: 'Certified pre-owned'.

Rebecca: 'Some original parts.'

I wonder what my Blue Book value is now.

Only the one chest tube, and a wrist IV in case it's suddenly needed. When they remove a tube, they literally spread spackle in the hole and slap on a dressing.

It was likely hydrogel, which is mostly water, glorified Vaseline (according to my charming C/T Surgery doctor; she was the only one they ever sent to do it), and some other doctory stuff, to encourage healing and prevent infection. You scoop it out of a foil packet and slather it into the incision/wound/hole/asteroid crater, then cover it with the adhesive bandage. That might be impregnated with medical goodness, too. Comes in a self-contained kit.

Me: "Bio-Spackle. Ask for it by name wherever fine medical and torture devices are sold."

Julie: We want a pic of said spackle (suspicious eyes).

Google 'wound dressing kit' and your prayer shall be answered.

Maria: So, have you picked out your Borg name yet?

Me: "Doofus of Borg."

Failed TV sitcom: 'Borg and Mindy.'

4/16/19
Yeah, I got transplanted during National Donate Life Month. Got first diagnosis of possible amyloid during Amyloidosis Month. I'm a cliché.

Too bad that turned out to be moot. But guess which month is also, conveniently, Sarcoidosis Month?

I hope there's no such thing as Slow Disembowelment Month.

Looks like I may actually get out of this hospital today, 8 days after the heart transplant and the 17th day in health-jail. Still a fingers-crossed situation, though.

Rebecca: I know you are ready, but is your wife ready?

Me: Absolutely not.

Janet: Exciting and terrifying for me, too. I've been alone in our house with the dog since Friday night and it is not a healthy thing to have long conversations with a basset hound. I want him to come home, but I'm terrified that something will happen and we'll need to rush back. I made it to the HR office and Safeway with my impaired eyesight and didn't hit anything. Getting down to Anshutz would be suicidal. I need to have a bunch of folks who can be there for transport duty in a pinch. There will be once-a-week biopsies for the first month and every other week for a few more months starting next week. Not sure of the schedule yet.

Something about this combination of meds makes me easily weepy at sentimental stuff. THAT'S gonna confuse the hell out of everybody who's spent more than five minutes around me.

It went away as soon as I got home. Coincidence? I think not.

Janet: Weepy and cranky both. It's the steroids, most likely. My mom on steroids was a roller- coaster for both of us. My dad on steroids was really hungry.

Terry W.: With all the things you've gone through, you need recovery time. Don't expect too much of yourself right away (I know this advice is too late — I've seen you prancing around on FB). Just telling you.

Liana: I've heard it is a common post-op temporary situation.

I was in mourning for my lost heart. Then, when I saw the pictures of the zombie artifact, it was all "Get thee behind me, Satan!"

Julie: From over here it seemed like you were prepping for the worst. Now, really through no action on your part, you have the best. I'd be all weepy, too.

Last chest drain just removed, the ginormous long one next to the heart, with a collection bottle at my knee. Getting that yanked out was a special experience. But I'm now tethered to only the one wrist IV, though they aren't putting anything into it.

I swear the thing was longer than the sandworms in 'Dune'. She literally pulled hand-over-hand for what seemed like 20 minutes.

You have to take a deep breath and hum while it's coming out. Apparently, the pressure makes it easier and hurt less. Or maybe the medical world just wants to encourage basic musicianship in the transplant community.

You'll notice I didn't make a 'hummer' joke. My new heart is more mature than that, apparently.

Just walked a mile with no chest tubes in. Seemed about as fast a pace as before the surgery, so that last long drain was probably interfering with breathing a little. But it does feel like a baby alien blasted out of me.

Which isn't far from the truth, though it had a whole birthing team.

Maria: You still have to breathe. I know it hurts, but you have to. Suffocated purple is not a good color on anyone.

Ladies and gentlemen, you are looking at a guy about to leave the hospital 8 days after his heart transplant. Biopsy negative. The paperwork is being processed as we speak. Homeward bound.

Janet: Yay!

Dave: You're about to get mugged by bassets!!!

Jeff: And Terry has left the building!

Meds. Not all of them yet, either. (photo 43)

Janet: Wow.

Erin: So in the UK, instead of a bunch of bottles, you would get a giant blister pack that have your pills for the day grouped in each blister. (It gets adjusted by the "chemist" as needed). That way you aren't fighting with bottles, and you easily know which pills you've taken for the day. (If you have multiple per day pills, again it's still organized via the blister pack) And there is your random factoid for the day.

Not sure that would've worked for me, as my meds and dosages did a lot of changing, especially at first (still being adjust, actually). The bottles let me add or subtract a certain amount without needing a new trip to the pharmacy.

Sarah: You're going to need a big pill box!

Barbara: Wow! And a whole bunch of instructions, too.

Julie: You're going to need a pill-sorter thingie.

Me: Have 2 already. They fit.

I would like to proudly announce that I am wearing actual clothes for the first time in 2 1/2 weeks. Underwear is NOT overrated.

*Despite the fact that you've all been overwhelmed by my bold fashion choice of ass-baring tablecloth and rumpled smiley-face socks, those absolutely are **not** considered clothing by* *most sentient beings.*

Apparently, there's a big transplant ceremony where I have ring to a silver bell and make a speech for surviving this. Between the circumstances and the steroids, I figure I'll last about 3 words.

Jacqueline: "I'm Not Dead" should do it.

Me: I'm not dead YET."

Jacqueline: That's four words. Concision is everything.

Melanie: "I got better!"

Scott: Asking YOU to make a speech? They don't know what they're in for, do they?

Dave: "So long Muthaf**kers!" It's right up there with Shakespeare!

I believe I'll eschew that sort of language toward people who may be called upon to revive me later.

Sean: I would reach for the bell, clutch my chest, and sink to my knees. Then start laughing. They might kill you, but what a way to go.

I like the way you think.

Kelly: So what'd you say? Did anyone film it?

Me: Just had to read words off of the wall.

I am in the car and we are outta here, baby! #hospitaljailbreak

Janet: Woo-hoo!!!!!

Cameron: So is that 9 days post-transplant? That's nuts!

8, actually. But your opinion is still valid

To access the photos/videos/links:
www.terrykroenungink.com/246-2/

5) Leaving Lost Vagus

4/16-4/30/19

This bit covers the event-filled first 2 weeks home, when I was adjusting to sleeping in my own bed for 8 hours at a time. Literally the only time that had happened in the preceding 2 ½ weeks had been when I was out cold during the actual transplant surgery. Not a recommended way to get your 40 winks, by the way. Mama Fentanyl will take your soul.

I learned that being able to actually stand under a steamy shower gives steamy sex a run for its money.

I also learned that managing all of the exotic medications requires a PhD in Astrophysics and the predictive skill of Nostradamus' smarter sister.

I was slow, achy, med-woozy, exhausted, and getting off the couch took a team of Clydesdales.

Fun fact: my grandpa once got to drive the real Budweiser Clydesdale team and wagon. (Bud, you do owe me some benjamins for that product placement)

By the end of April I was walking 5K at a time at 17 minutes per mile. To hear the doctors and my Facebook crew talk about it, this was as miraculous as an armadillo standing on its hind legs and dancing the 'Macarena' while smoking weed. I'll have to take their word on that.

Fun fact: armadillos are the only creature on earth to get leprosy, besides humans.

At the end of this part my mom, brother, and sister fly in to visit the tragic patient. Despite my living in America's vacation destination for 21 years, this is the first time any of them had come here to see us. If I'd known how easy it would be to get them on the plane, I'd have tried to die ages ago.

Oh…and I resumed proper pooping. I know you were worried about that.

4/16/19
First heart-healthy meal out of the hospital: cheeseburger & fries from McDonald's. #justagaglightenup

FYI, haters: the doctors let me have hamburgers while in the Cardiac ICU post-transplant.

Well, it was no bison meatloaf, but it hit the spot, nonetheless.

Maria: Lunch of champions!

Scott: It's what 19-year-olds eat!

Alaena: That's what I said. Heart: "Finally some real food!"

Courtney: Clog those new arteries!

Me: Believe me, it was a one-time thing. Normally I eat like an Olympic runner. Other than a couple of items, like grapefruit, that interfere with immunosuppression, the doctors said I should eat my normal healthy runner's diet.

Matthew: After my two surgeries earlier this year, my wife asked me what I wanted to do about dinner, and I said, "Taco Bell!"

Good call. Eventually they'll win the Franchise Wars (according to that essential work of near-Nostradamian futurism, 1993's 'Demolition Man').

PL: Good for you. Some people just don't realize how wonderful normalcy is, and a burger and fries says it all. After my husband's brain surgery, and months in the hospital/care center, that is what he wanted as well.

I'm sitting on my own couch, in my own house, after having my first proper bath in nearly 3 weeks.

Nearly had to hire a sandblasting crew to get the grunge off.

Veronica: Living the dream.

Deborah: Click your heels together, and repeat after me, "There's no place like home!"

If I'd thought that actually worked, I'd have been a heel-clicking madman a long time before. But red's just not my color. And pumps? Puuuhleeze!

Judith: Nothing like that first shower/bath after surgery.

Julia: Terry, you going to stay home for a few weeks before you get back on your bike?

Me: Oh, yeah. That may be a late June thing.

It was quite a while before I could lean on my arms at all. 12 weeks before being officially cut loose to try a push-up.

Get a heart transplant, they said. All the cool kids are doing it, they said. (photo 44)

Christine: Just say no...to the random deposition of amyloid proteins in vital organs!

Alaena: Your new leash to the medical industrial complex.

Me: All labeled with a sharpie on top as to when and how many every day, then deposited in the morning bin, the evening bin, or both.

Eric: Holy #%$! So if you lived in the UK and if there were a no deal Brexit, you'd have to hurry up and learn Canadian, eh?

Christine: A heart transplant is not for the faint of heart...oh, wait. You've got this!

Me: Most of these are to counteract the nasty side effects of the anti-rejection meds, especially the Prednisone. But they hope to phase out the Prednisone soon and then some of the others will also go away.

Maria: You might need one of those pill towers instead of the flat boxes — I think this needs a three-dimensional distribution matrix.

Cindi: Good to know you can look forward to getting off the Prednisone — that stuff is no fun. But considering the alternative...

They started tapering me off of the Pred after 8 weeks. By August 1 I was only on half the original dose. Hands still shook like leaves in a gale, so it wasn't much help there.

Curtis: Wow. That is a lot of pills.

Me: Only 3 keep my heart from being rejected. Most of the rest are to counteract their nasty side effects, or are antibiotics to forestall the infections I can't fight now.

And a couple are just to tone down my sexy so I can safely walk down the street.

(Janet) First night home after first shower since the 30th of March. New shirt. New heart. A ton of meds. The shirt is Rosebud the Basselope from Berkeley Breathed's *Bloom County*. (photo 45)

Janet: He's very tired this morning as the reality of no uninterrupted sleep, the tons of puncture wounds, and the new heart routines set in.

Rebecca: His color is so good. It is amazing what a new heart can do. I know it is a long road, but hang in there.

It's my favorite shade, invented by the Elizabethans: 'Dying Spaniard', although 'Goose Turd Green' was a close second. Those are real colors, BTW.

AE: You look REALLY good! Eight days after childbirth, I still looked like a truck had run me over. They take a saw to your chest, rip out your heart, shove another one in and look at you! Next, you'll be tap dancing on the table. You absolutely amaze me.

You don't want to see that. I have the rhythm of a spastic camel. YouTube 'the Nicholas Brothers' instead. You'll thank me.

David: I've occasionally told people "Have a heart," but you took it way beyond most.

Me: Recycling: I walk the walk.

Sharon: I am positive that your absolute zest for life, your irreverence (which I admire, but cannot pull off), and your deep reservoir of I'm-going-to-pull-through-this-stuff (faith, whether you're religious or not) is 99% of the reason you're at home tonight. Yay! So happy for you and your wife, who may get a good night's sleep now. May the healing continue. Live long and prosper.

And 'Star Trek' gets referenced again. Woo-hoo!

More useless but fascinating info: the hand gesture Spock uses with that saying was adopted by Leonard Nimoy because it's close to the letter shin in Hebrew. His childhood rabbi used it to represent God at services.

Janet: As the novelty is starting to wear off and the reality of all the drugs and labs and trying vainly to find someone to help out with appointments setting in, (with well wishes being much appreciated, but the brass tacks of how to actually make this happen eluding us), we are both worn out and stressed. This is not a "Gee, you got a new heart and now go on your merry way" kind of thing. There's a team at the hospital to take care of Terry, but only me and my daughter struggling to do the rest. We'll make it work, somehow. We have to.

They both deserve some sort of award for it. Maybe just a parade down Pennsylvania Avenue and a simple 130-foot-tall monument.

Diane: I thought I was bad with 10 meds a day! You've got me beat! I hope they all help you stay healthy and strong for a long, long time!

4/17/19
About to post a photo of the full glorious horror of my transplant-ravaged torso. It'll be in the comments, so as to not surprise the unwilling. You are warned. #oversharingagain (photo 46)

Just a brief preview of my eventual autopsy pics.

Me: Big vertical line is where they opened me up with a car jack (only a little hyperbole). Shoulder staples are from removing the pacemaker. Everything else is from drainage tubes and temporary pacemaker wires. Notice how many there are. Those were all yanked out about every other day, while I had to grit my teeth and hum. Lots of bruising, but not at the main incision.

Jennifer: You know, not as bad as I thought it might be! That vertical scar is pretty gorgeous as far as scars go. Should hopefully heal up nicely.

Liana: All you need are some screws sticking out the side of your neck!

America kept requesting that, and who was I to disagree?

Me: Only hurts when coughing.

Or getting out of bed. Or getting into bed. Or turning over in bed. Or laughing. Or sneezing. Or...

Me: I look like a machine-gun victim on a slab at the morgue.

Maria: You could audition for all the corpse role on all the various *NYPD* spinoffs.

"What happened here, Sarge?"

"An ugly thing, Lieutenant. He stood up at a women's rights panel and said, 'Well, actually...'"

Rebecca: Nah, you have too much color in your face.

Sharon: In the words of some hero in a movie, " Chicks dig scars, glory last forever. " You look healthy.

Karen: Such a straight line! Did they use a ruler?

Me: Wouldn't be surprised. Accuracy is pretty essential in this business.

Eileen: I'm a trauma nurse in a family of medical people. We consider that dinner conversation. Bring it.

The wife was talking to the hospital that put in my pacemaker 2 years ago, to inform them of the situation and that they need no longer monitor a non-existent device. When she mentioned the surgeon who did my transplant, Dr. Fullerton, they spoke of him in the hushed reverent tones reserved for saints. Apparently, he's some sort of surgical demi-god here and nationally. Good to know that they went with the Hall of Fame pitcher.

Maria: I told you before — that's exactly what we all wanted for you, and not some junior burger cook named Bubba.

And once again, an unknowing public cruelly disparages Bubba's skills.

Currently 5'11", 152 lbs. Went into the hospital March 31 at 164. #brutalexperience #I'mabouttoblowaway

And I ate like a starving crocodile the whole time I was in there, too.

Julia: Not a good way to lose weight.

Bill: It that what they mean by having a "heavy heart?"

Maria: Lose another 50 and you can be a supermodel!

I look awful in fake angel wings, though.

Julie: You need pie.

Jay: Wow! You had a 12-pound heart!?

So this an actual thing: The Transplant Games of America.

Do they give you the medal, or does it go to the new heart?

Things you learn when they swap out your heart: the bacteria that causes annoying yeast infections is potentially fatal to me now, so I have to rinse my mouth 4 times a day with yellow goo to keep my

organs from being wrecked by it.

Yana: Yup, oral health is really important in transplants and they talk about it in the pre-transplant class. I remember of a case they wouldn't bump a woman on the liver transplant list until she quit smoking and fixed her teeth. They're not going to waste an organ if that person's habits were going to make it fail anyway. Is it flavored at least?

Me: Not bad, as medicines go. There's banana in it.

Mark: What's the name of the yellow goo?

Me: Nystatin.

Mark: I've had them as tablets. What have they advised for maintaining general gut health? I've found it can throw your gut balance out if you're on them for a while.

Me: Haven't mentioned that yet. With the other antibiotics they give you, the microbiome is probably pretty thin forever.

Mark: Fermented foods are the gem I've found. Saurkraut and the like. Instead of introducing millions of bugs with pills or yoghurt, fermented foods create a very friendly environment for your own natural good bacteria to thrive. Seems to work better for me, anyway, as the pill forms of fresh biotics I've found upset my gut, too, but the fermentations are gentler and long-term work for me way better. Ask about it anyway, next chat you have with the docs. Head off any problems before they start.

Cindi: Oh, that stuff is gross. I had chronic yeast infections for a while (in my vocal cords) and had to use that Nystatin stuff. I shuddered on your behalf when I read this post.

(Meme) "I don't feel like I'm getting older. It's more like my warranty has expired and my parts are wearing out."

But, at least, I have a 100,000-mile service plan on my new motor. When I eventually check out, they'll have to beat that heart to death with a stick.

4/18/19
Another little post-transplant joy: getting up at 6:15 am to drive to the hospital for a blood draw at 7.

Christine: How long is that going to continue?

Me: Looks like a weekly thing, halfway to forever.

That one turned out to be just a one-off, thankfully.

Christine: Well, weekly is better than daily. Hugs!

Me: This is local, so it's not the end of the world. But we also have to drive 60 minutes to the medical center weekly for a month, then bi-weekly, until they're happy about rejection odds.

Barbara: How come they don't send nurses to the house to draw?

For the same reason we don't get house calls from doctors: insurance company BS.

Maria: Can't you just bite your own vein and FedEx it to them in a jar?

I had to do this with a stool sample. I've had better days.

Veronica: I feel like they already took enough.

Yeah, they owe me some. Maybe a tanker truck will back up to the house with my change.

Me: They took so much in the hospital that they had to give me iron through my IV.

That looked like blood going in, actually.

Sarah: I hope you survive the recovery process! My mom had to do weekly IV's for 6 months. Her nurse told her to start eating dark chocolate right before her appointments to help with the sticks. She says it helped. Plus, chocolate.

Ana: Can they draw it at Longs Peak and have them send it over?

Me: That's what we did.

Sheila: Bet you're fasting, too.

Me: Not for this one. Can't eat Tuesday before the biopsy, though, since sedation is involved.

Just woke up from a nap, because I was having a dream about being in the African bush in the 19th century, taking orders from village chiefs for Girl Scout cookies. WTF? Not sure what they put in these post-transplant meds.

Harriet: But were they made of real Girl Scouts?

Me: Perhaps. Just like they make baby oil.

Sheila: Good drugs!

I'm sure you were all hovering over FB waiting to hear that my tacrolimus trough number is now perfect. #antirejectionmed

Julia: Not sure what a tacrolimus trough is, but perfect sounds good.

The main rejection med they monitor. The trough is the lowest amount in my system, 12 hours after taking it and immediately before the next dose. They want a certain level at that point as a floor.

Cal: Does that mean BP and heart rate are excellent?

Me: It means I'm absorbing that anti-rejection drug like I should, which means it's doing its job. In the hospital it started off at 2 and they were mildly concerned that it might be an issue.

It soon got up to the desired 12-13. By early July it had dropped so much (8.8, very low normal) that they had to boost the dosage. By late July my white cell count was dangerously low and the transplant team went into emergency mode. But they couldn't overdo that, as my white blood cell count was in the basement and any more immunosuppression would totally crash it. This is all an art as much as a science.

Just did my first outdoor walk with the new heart. Half a mile at most, at the speed of the basset hound we were 'exercising', but it was a walk.

Maria: I am sure the basset hound was perfectly happy.

Hard to tell. They always look like miserable little poops on their way to the guillotine.

Walked a mile outdoors around our entire development, unattended, in 18:50. Not terribly slower than I was doing it before all of this happened. Nothing hurt, though the Frankenstein chest was tight and needs to be gradually stretched out. Hurts more turning over in bed, actually.

Cal: I would think you would have to sleep on your back, yes?

Me: Today I've managed side sleeping. Research told me it wouldn't damage anything, so long as it didn't hurt.

I'm pretty much a constant right-side sleeper, so finally being able to do that instead of being on my back, elevated, for 3 weeks made me a happy camper.

4/19/19
Looks like I was premature on the post-surgical bruising. Now half my chest has turned green and the thigh next to one femoral artery is a spectacular maroon the size of my palm.

Julia: In other words, you look like a rainbow.

♬ *"Look, look, follow the rainbow; follow the fellow who follows our dream."*

And that, my friends, is the allusion to the obscure 1946 Broadway musical 'Finian's Rainbow,' about leprechauns and Southern racism, that you've been expecting all this while. You're welcome.

Liana: As long as they're not bright red, you're good.

You know, there's a certain relieved liberation in no longer having to pee into a plastic bottle while over-worked ladies stare at you doing it.

Though if I'd kept backing away from the bottle each time while hollering, "Let's go for the distance record, babes!", that would've at least been entertaining. Well, not so much for the housekeeping staff.

Julia: Showoff.

Maria: You mean you didn't enjoy having your own personal urinal harem?

That was the alternative title for this book.

Janus: You need to write a book about your heart transplant.

Maria: TOTALLY!

Christine: I actually want Terry and Janet to write the book, alternating chapters from their alternating viewpoints of the situation.

Okay, okay! Enough with the nagging. Here we are. Happy now?

Sharon: And make a production out of it?

Jim: With song and dance numbers!

Can't. Somebody already wrote 'Urinetown.'

If you aren't musical savvy, that's an actual Broadway show. Maybe it's on the Internet somewhere and you can, um, live stream it.

Sarah: You can even pee with the door shut!

Russell: Trump would pay good money to do that.

Walked a mile twice today, the second in 18 minutes, and closed the exercise rings on the Apple watch. 9,000 steps, 4.2 miles of moving, while wearing my new apparel item. (photo 47)

And thus began my collection of smart-assed transplant shirts. Next I'll collect transplant thongs.

Sweet mother of Odin, acid reflux after a heart transplant is all the tortures of the seven hells of the damned. 3 hours! And a couple hours later, it came back. #longnight #90minutesfeltlike90years

On the floor in a fetal position crying, that's how bad it was. Eventually those went away, so I'm thinking it was a combination of still-very-much-raw inner tissues and the stomach adjusting to the awful meds.

Me: At first, I thought the new heart was dying, that's how much it hurt. But when Pepcid and Pepto toned it down a tiny bit, briefly, I knew it was 'only' acid burning unhealed tissue. #noteagerforarepeat

Re: 'only acid': Stomach acid is hydrochloric acid, potassium chloride, and sodium chloride. It has the same ph as battery acid and will corrode metal. You make 1.5 liters of the stuff **a day***. The only reason it doesn't eat completely through you and go all the way to China like the xenomorph blood in 'Alien' is that your stomach also makes bicarbonate (a base, the opposite of an acid) to neutralize the excess, and it makes a mucous lining as a buffer.*

Another horrifying fun fact: potassium chloride is the drug they use in lethal injections to **cause cardiac arrest***.*

Alaena: What did you eat?

Me: Salad, bread, cheese, veggie chicken nuggets. I blame the last.

Stephany: Might also be related to all the walking today.

Me: Walked after dinner, so maybe.

Russell: Chicken nuggets? Are you mad?

You're not wrong, on so many levels.

Jill: At least there's a healthy heart in there to feel the burn for you.

Joe: Start taking Prilosec every morning, at least until you're healed. I had to do the same thing.

Me: They already have me on reflux meds as part of my zillion pills a day. Not impressed.

Mark: Green tea and licorice. Check first about the licorice, it can affect blood pressure.

Cal: I literally wrote the book *The Healing Powers of Tea.* Did you know some chamomile teas contain licorice & can cause a spike in BP?

Alaena: Green tea maybe, nope on licorice (pretty much no herbs or supplements that haven't been studied specifically for contradiction with the anti-rejection meds).

Mark: Yeah, I've found green tea alone a big help with acid.

Me: We eat absurdly healthy. Always have. Wife's a vegetarian, which means I mostly am.

Cal: Ditto. On occasion I force myself 2 eat fish or poultry 4 the protein...but vegetarian/vegan – go back and forth.

Me: What's most annoying is that they have me on reflux meds (Protonix).

Ana: The reflux meds did nothing for me, so I finally saw Sarah and she recommended some bitters (yucky, but did it). Plus cutting down on the acidic foods, especially before bedtime.

Sarah: Bitters, 15 minutes before you eat. Helps the body remember when it is supposed to create more acid.

Cindi: The acid reflux could be a side effect of your meds. I have to take medicine every day for acid reflux, because it's terrible even when your heart has not just recently been removed and replaced! You may want to put that in your daily regimen of meds. You can get it over the counter but you can also get it from a prescription so whichever way is cheaper for you. I would just ask your doctors to be sure it doesn't interfere with any of your meds.

Me: GERD meds are already part of what they have taking every day.

4/20/19
And this is what I get to wear whenever I leave the house. As fashionable as it is sexy. (photo 48)

Cheri: That'll be a lifesaver, but when I saw A POS, I'm not gonna lie, the first thing I thought of was "A piece of s***."

No, you're thinking of my stool sample.

Cheri: What does A POS stand for, anyway?

Alaena: A Positive blood type.

Aimie: Sexy AF, bro!

Veronica: Trés chic.

AE: Veeeery cool indeed! They might want to chip you next.

I can have it done at my dog's vet on her next appointment.

Mandy: A badge of honour as a survivor.

So I'm the one with the near-death experience, but it's my wife who just a notice in the mail saying, "You may qualify for a state program to pay your final expenses."

Headline: "Pothole may have saved man's life by jolting heart back into normal rhythm." (link #4)

It would've been nice if my problem could've been fixed so easily.

See? This is why you shouldn't get those shocks fixed on your car.

Tomorrow's Easter Sunday and 2 weeks since my surgical resurrection, make of that what you will.

Alaena: Happy Necromancy Day?

Maria: You are the best-looking zombie I've ever known.

> ♫ *'Back to back, ghoul, belly to belly,*
> *Well, I don't give a damn 'cause I'm stone dead already,*
> *Back to back, oh oh oh, belly to belly,*
> *It's a zombie jamboree.'*

4/21/19
You know your life has changed when you have to take osteoporosis meds because your other meds destroy your bones.

"Look at the bones!" — Tim the Enchanter, reacting to a certain killer rabbit

Me: Plus ginormous calcium/vitamin D pills twice a day.

Christine: Can I be glad you still have a life to change? Post-mortem decomposition would have played havoc with your bones as well.

Actually, those suckers will probably still be around come the Last Judgement.

In honor of the 2nd weekiversary of the new heart, I just managed to walk 2 miles non-stop in 33:57, which is 16:55 a mile (better than 3.5 mph). Pretty close to what I would've walked it before all of this happened. Sucking wind, because all of my conditioning evaporated (along with 13 pounds I couldn't afford to lose; I weigh 152 lbs. right now) in the past few weeks. Things are nicely on track.

Jim: You can be Death for Comic-Con.

"The salmon mousse!" (yet another Monty Python quote, from 'The Meaning of Life')
(link #5)

Great. Now the staples are itching like crazy. I know that's a good thing, but...

Alaena: Get a hair dryer with a cool air setting. Sometime blowing a little air in it can hold off the itch.

(gritting teeth: "No blow job jokes, no blow job jokes...")

Siobahn: We used vitamin E oil to help with the itch and healing the skin. Lavender oil works, too.

What about vitamin Wonka? (look that one up yourself; I'm on a deadline here)

Janus: Don't scratch and don't put anything on them, it will promote skin growth. You don't want your skin to grow over the staples.! Take it from me, I just had thirty removed.

Regarding the recent weight loss because of all this: I can literally wrap my thumb and little finger around my wrist.

*I can get my thumb and middle finger around my **ankle**.*

Me: I have tiny bones and the wrists were always a joke, but still...

Cerene: Pfft! Go eat a sammich, Skeletor!

The damaged right wrist, the one that turned purple from all of the IV's, is mostly clear of the bruising, but now it's decided to hurt when I move it.

Jim: It'll have to come out.

I have a spare.

Transplanted hearts bang away at more BPM than regular hearts, due to various complicated surgical reasons, like having no vagus nerve anymore. Mine runs around 100 for normal purposes. It also

seems to only drop to about 83, even in the dead of night, snoring. It does that when I sit for a long time, too, which is why I have to get up and walk around every now and then when on the couch or else I'll fall asleep. When the pacemaker was in, it had a bottom setting of 50 and I felt the same as at 88 now.

If I sit too long my head spins for a second when I stand up, as Archie McThump-Thump takes longer to react to movement now. Teenagers, lazy slobs, am I right?

Julie: Will that change ever, or is it a thing now?

Me: That's likely it, but we won't know until everything heals and I can get back to regular biking, running, etc.

Cal: Curious about your age? Late 50s, early 60s?

Me: Just turned 61 before all of this. But I'm a 'Colorado 61', so my over-exercised body tracks lots younger, according to the doctors.

I count 50 staples in my abused corpus. I bet those will be an unfettered joy to have removed in May.

Max: Don't stand in the microwave, those are gonna arc like CRAZY.

Scott: Well, the unfettered part is right...

David: You should definitely try a TSA line or two before they come out.

They'd spend 20 minutes making me take off my shoes/belt and wondering why the machine still beeped.

Shae: My son had 45 removed, thanks to a pit bull attack. He said it was all painless...the staple removal that is...not the attack. Hopefully, it will be painless for you, too.

It was. About the only painless thing in this whole dreary mess.

24 pills a day. This is not hyperbole.

Jacqueline: Hyper-pill-e?

Serge: That's a bitter pill to swallow. ("Not just one.")

Julia: I only take 11, plus 5 shots.

4/22/19
The ugly green delayed bruising is making the chest ache and making me work a bit harder to breathe.

Kelly: Is that normal?

Me: Probably.

Sarah: I know you want another pill like a hole in the head, but homeopathic Arnica is amazing for bruising and it will not affect your meds.

Homeopathic Arnica? Isn't she the sister of Negasonic Teenage Warhead?

Me: I have to have all meds and supplements approved by my Transplant Team.

Janet: The doctors were adamant that nothing be mixed with the 20 meds he takes, especially botanicals, mostly because there hasn't been enough testing to determine the reactions. They have the final say.

Maria: It's not easy being green.

Veronica: I find naming the bruise helps, because you have a name to curse at. I suggest Bruise Wayne.

I prefer Bruise Banner. You won't like me when I'm 'hangry.'

Or, since it was royally annoying and I felt like hollering "Great Scot!" every time I looked at it, Robert the Bruise.

Though I might go with Lenny Bruise, since 'socially inappropriate comedian' is sort of my brand.

Putting all of my heart-related FB posts onto one document. There may be a book in this, a short one. Might have to print it in 64-point type.

A short one? Hahahaha!!! (this manuscript is 279 pages right now, and I have 70 pages to add snark to, yet)

Me: 12 pages of posts, only up to Day 1 in the hospital in Denver.

Sharon: Your journey would be inspiring for others on a similar path.

Mark: *Diary of a Heart Transplant, or, Tis but a Scratch.*

Karen: You should make a graphic novel out of it.

Oh, it's pretty graphic, alright. Wait till you see the pictures of the dead heart. You'll wish it was only radio.

Back to the hospital tomorrow for a biopsy, more tests, and a chat with the guy who slapped in the new heart. A weekly thing for a while as they watch for rejection. Just your typical observance of Shakespeare's birthday.

AE: Don't forget to give the guy who slapped in the new hearty a slap on the back for job well done.

Eileen: There's got to be an appropriate Shakespeare quote for that. If I were smarter, I'd have it.

"Vengeance is in my heart, death in my hand/ Blood and revenge are hammering in my head." – Aaron, 'Titus Andronicus'

Then they buried him alive. It doesn't pay to talk smack to Romans.

Can't take my morning meds tomorrow until after the blood draw, so I'm taking them to the biopsy appointment in a baggie with a picture of Thanos on it. #appropriate

The biopsy was a, um, snap.

Tim: Check with the Transplant Team. I think the only one you need to hold is the tac. At least that's what they have me doing anytime labs are drawn.

Me: True, but it's less confusing to just bag them all.

Tim: What time is your appointment? What time do you usually take your morning meds?

Me: They asked us to go with 8 a.m. and 8 p.m., since it would simplify their morning tac trough tests on clinic days. That won't work when I teach again, though. Have to go earlier. But by then we should be down to just monthly clinics/biopsies.

Transplant rejection meds have to be taken twice a day, twelve hours apart. That's how we live our lives, half a day at a time. My Apple watch nags me.

Tim: Do you have them go through the neck while awake?

Honestly, why would you want that needle anywhere else?

Me: With supposedly light anesthesia. Last week they overdid it and I was hung over for 6 hours like a bad Mardi Gras weekend. Today I'll get them to tone it down.

Me: They barely gave me any today. Much better. Awake the whole time, no after-effects. Next week we won't bother with it.

The nurse actually said, "You're a lightweight." Like Dorothy Parker said, "One more drink and I'll be under the host."

She also said, "If all the young ladies who attended the Yale promenade dance were laid end to end, no one would be the least surprised."

Tim: I didn't use any because I wanted to get back home ASAP. It's not that bad. Soon it will be every other week. Then every 4 - 6 weeks. I have my next biopsy on 5/1 along with the AlloMap. The one after that with another AlloMap. If both tests show similar results, I will only have biopsies annually with AlloMaps every 8 weeks.

Now I do them with no anesthetic except Lidocaine at the catheter site. I get to be a smartass while they do it and no forced recovery time. In fact, they have me walk to the Cath Lab and I walk out re-dressed and check out from there straight to the car.

AlloMap is a genetic blood test for rejection, so you don't have to endure biopsies. You have to be stable and have a history of no rejection first, so it isn't done right after the transplant.

3 sneezes in 5 seconds. My chest pillow was in another room. #ouch

AE: No, no, no — you go nowhere without that damn pillow!

90 lbs. of pressure on a sawn sternum. Yum…

4/23/19
Maria sent me a stuffed Cerberus. This hospital is literally Hell. (photo 49)

Mandy: You got a Spot!!

Maria: It's not just any Spot. It's a Squishable Spot.

Correction: it's a Fluffy (Hagrid's 3-headed dog in 'Harry Potter').

Aimie: Hey! And he'd make a suitable cough pillow if the official one isn't handy!!!

Yes, it did, though I had to squish the air out of it first.

Garalt: I pictured Hades' guardian somewhat less huggable.

About to meet with the transplant nurse practitioner who supposedly has the photos of my old dead heart. So this full day at the hospital may not be a total waste.

Alaena: Now we get to speculate how you were still alive. It really was that bad.

'Natural contrariness' has the best odds. 'The Afterlife wants nothing to do with him' is a close second.

Just saw the pictures of my old heart, cut open. Holy hell, it's a wonder I lived to get to the hospital. Completely full of growths, walls so thick they couldn't pump, sarcoid crowding out most of the walls. If you knew nothing about hearts, you could still tell it was useless.

Right ventricle at left. The 3 slices stack on top of one another. Everything white is the bad stuff. The other photo is what it's supposed to look like. (photo 50, 51)

No self-respecting zombie would've tolerated this thing. It would be below his standards.

Carrie: So glad for the new heart!

Sarah: What is the next step for amyloid/sarcoidosis prevention? Or is there?

Me: Low dose of Prednisone prevents the sarcoidosis.

5 mg, they tell me.

Jeffrey: What a weird experience it must be to see something like that...our ancestors wouldn't have been able to conceive of it.

Daniel: Looks like a foreskin collection.

Looks like the failed practice attempts of a student mohel (that's what the ritual circumciser is called in Judaism; trust me, you want a guy with experience for this).

FYI, you really can't live long with a pump that looks like this. The doctors can't believe I was still upright and functioning. #that'sareallynecessarytransplant

All of the white is the bad infiltrative stuff, crowding out healthy heart cells. And the walls themselves are much too thick, making them inelastic so the heart can't pump.

Carrie: Holy shit! Do they think this was starting back when you got the pacemaker?

'Holy shit!' is literally what every medical professional says when they see the photo.

Me: Yeah. They said at the time that I was too young for a pacemaker, but nobody looked too hard because the echocardiogram was still normal.

Karen: Holy F! It's amazing you didn't die!

Me: Literally true, they said.

Veronica: Holy shit.

Eileen: Crikey.

Linda: Wow. It has got to be weird to look at slices of your own former heart. Now that's an experience very few of us will ever have!

Me: There's a hospital in Houston that'll let you HOLD it.

Sarah: Taking a broken heart to a whole new level.

Chris: I can't stop myself asking a potentially ignorant question. Now that you have a 19-year-old heart, are you going to live to be the oldest man ever?

Me: I wish. All of the rest of me is still 61.

Jacqueline: Thank God for modern medicine! #mostnecessarytransplantever

Kelly: Jesus!!! Are they trying to find out what causes this disease?

Me: They sent samples off to the Mayo Clinic for exotic analysis.

Cal: How did you know you had heart issues? Bloodwork showing high cholesterol? Out of breath? High BP?

Me: Out of breath for no reason. Couldn't sustain talking while walking. Occasional chest pains.

Brandt: Looks like a badly cooked pork medallion.

Marisa: Wow. I kinda wanted a picture of your heart before it was cut into pieces.

Me: I believe it was a judicial execution of the heart for attempted murder.

Garalt: This is just astonishing given how fit you were and how many miles you went on those two wheels. Wow.

And that, folks, is how you properly observe Shakespeare's birthday, by observing a heart so tragic that even Iago and Richard III would buy you a beer to help you recover from the shock.

All done with the second biopsy. I had them crank down the sedation to almost non-existent, to avoid the 6-hour hangover I had last time. Awake all the way. It took far longer for the nurses to prep me than for the doctor to run catheters into my heart and take samples. That was only about 10 minutes.

Ali: Where did they put the tube in? Or did they leave a port for it?

Me: Neck again. Jugular vein. They just numbed it and poked a new hole.

*FYI: the jugular vein drains deoxygenated blood out if the brain/ head and back to the heart via the superior vena cava (which is about an inch in diameter). There is an inferior vena cava, but we don't have anything to do with **that** lowlife.*

Strolled back into the Cardiac ICU to give them a thrill. Everywhere I go here people marvel at the progress. Got a hug from one of the nurses who took care of me.

Transplants must go sideways with enough regularity that they get positively giddy when it doesn't. The team has made it very clear that I'm the exception, not the rule. Good to hear that.

It is weird that my simple pacemaker implantation was a messed-up horror show, but the full heart transplant was silky-smooth.

The 50 staples in my corpus come out in 2 weeks.

Ali: Think of all the sewing that saved them!

Ironically, Janet is a trained seamstress/fashion designer.

Me: Oh, they sewed their brains out. All of the heart vessels had to be connected with tiny unleaking sutures.

Eileen: And you can go as Frankenstein's buddy for Halloween.

I need to work on my performance of "Puttin' on the Ritz, then."

From Mel Brooks' seminal work of postmodern realism, 'Young Frankenstein.'

90 freaking minutes waiting past the appointment time and this doctor still hasn't shown up.

Me: I'll cut him some slack, since he did put the heart in, and said I can drive in a week.

He cut me open, I cut him slack…all even, right?

Sessha: The best docs are also the busiest docs. You are no longer critically ill (yay) so you will often have to wait while he deals with those that are (boo).

The transplant surgeon say I can drive in a week. Woo-hoo!

Maria: Did he say what you could drive?

Me: Drive everybody nuts, most likely.

Julia: I thought you had already done that.

Me: They originally said 6-8 weeks, until the sternum fully healed and an airbag wouldn't undo the surgery.

Julia: That is huge. But no bike riding.

Me: That'll be 8-12 weeks from transplant, so it's totally healed in case I fall off.

Week 8 I was back on that sucker. Got up to 25 miles at a time by Week 12. Some time I'll work my way up to climbing the local hill I call Mount Doom, which pitches up to a 14% gradient.

4/24/19
My skin cancer risk is now literally 1000% higher, so I can't go to the mailbox without SPF 250 an inch thick. So you might want to invest in sunblock stock. I'm personally about to raise their profits.

Maria: Is getting dipped in Teflon an option?

Me: Actually, they said SPF 30 is fine.

The protection difference between SPF 30 and SPF 50: 30 blocks 97% of the UV rays; 50 blocks 98%.

Julie: Is it a side effect of the meds?

Me: Yep. Suppressed immune system affects everything.

Cameron: Invest in some SPF clothing!

Beth: Yep...get SPF shirt, hat and pants. I wear the shirts when I run because I hate putting all the stuff on all the time. It's cheaper in the long run, too.

SPF goodies: I now have a long-billed ball cap, a long-sleeved breathable running shirt, a spectacularly ugly hiking hat with the brim all the way around, and a cycling jersey. The only thing missing from my collection is the coveted SPF mankini.

AE: A Spiderman suit would be easier.

Jeff: Suit of armor?

Chad: Black Sith Robes?

Wookie costume?

The pictures of my old heart look like slices of tomato you'd get on a BLT in Satan's Deli.

In the dumpster behind Satan's deli, actually.

Just walked 5 kilometers nonstop, about 17:40 a mile. 17th day after transplant.

(Janet) Our outing today to pick up meds and eat lunch proved to be more stressful than anticipated. Terry's prescriptions were sent to our local Safeway pharmacy but they couldn't fill them because the prescriptions were also sent to the hospital pharmacy and the insurance said no way are you getting refills so soon. Panic calls to the Transplant Team and calls to Safeway got Terry enough meds for a couple of days at least until the full amounts are filled. He has a strict every 12-hour schedule that if deviated from, can lead to rejection. This was scary.

This happened more than once. Now we only use the local hospital pharmacy, which is open 24/7 and is 5 minutes from our house. It's right next to the gift shop, whatever that might mean.

Me: And still I didn't have an autistic meltdown. #progress

The Wellbutrin seems to be working. Yesterday I felt a violent tantrum coming on, but then it just faded away. Easier on the furniture, and Janet's nerves, that way.

Alaena: Perhaps the increased oxygenated blood to your head is making you less testy?

I'm a teacher, I'm always 'testy.' Though sometimes I'm just 'quizzy.'

Maria: You know...isn't it highly advisable to keep transplant patients stress-free, relaxed, and happy? 'Cause I don't think they are doing it right.

They say I'm as stress-free as this gets, compared to everybody else.

2nd heart biopsy totally negative for rejection.

Angie: That's because you're a seasoned writer and seasoned writers are immune to rejection.

I don't know about immune. Resigned, maybe.

Maria: And Cerberus is doing his job keeping all the nasties away.

The cute and fuzzy nasties, yes.

11,000 steps today. Haven't been able to do that since March.

Maria: Amazing. Wanna come to Zumba next week?

Can't. I'm in a Brazilian ju-jitsu tournament. Then I have a powerlifting competition.

4/25/19
Another charming side effect of the transplant: my pre-existent pulsative tinnitus (permanent ringing in the ears that goes up in pitch with each heartbeat) is a LOT more noticeable, especially at night when it's quiet and there are no distractions. Sounds like a banshee when it's 100 beats per minute.

Constantly fighting it. A sort of tinnitussle.

Alaena: Play music before bed.

Tchaikovsky's '1812 Overture', so the ringing is barely noticeable in comparison?

Richard: I wish you wouldn't have shared that. Just the word makes me notice mine; it may be hours before my brain switches gears to ignore.
Liana: I just think of my tinnitus as the symphonic accompaniment to my life.

Concerto in D minor for Brain-Banshee and Flugelhorn. ♫ "I got the noise right here, it's shriekin' in your ear…"

Stephany: I am now on permanent blood thinners and they have made the ear-ringing my permanent soundtrack. My complaint is that the ringing used to be my only precursor to migraines, so now it sounds like I'm always about to get a headache. I'm working on reprogramming my expectations.

Julie: I bought an Alexa for the bedroom specifically so I can set what white sounds at whatever volume works without getting out of bed.

We use a fan for that. Seems to work. Janet says I can't have another woman in the bedroom.

Melisse: I have significant hearing loss in my tinnitus ear. A hearing aid has helped so much. I hear background sounds now that drown out the tinnitus.

Julie: It will be interesting to see if when you can run and bike ride and get the pulse rate down if it goes away.

DSA test came back on the heart for antibody rejection. Totally negative again. #cleanasawhistlesofar

I made my antibodies cry uncle.

Jeff: Keep being negative about this!

I positively will.

Grandkid took photos of dead heart to school for some sort of 10-year-old show-and-tell. I can only imagine the joyous response. #whowillsavethechildren?

Samantha: I once took a live black widow spider to show and tell in a peanut butter jar.

How'd you manage to fit yourself into a peanut butter jar?

Stephany: My son was given a very large rifle bullet, made with no gunpowder. Just because it's cool and the guy thought my son would like it. He did. He liked it so much he took it to school to show his friends. Then we had a lovely visit with the principal.

Cameron: Personally, I would have been asking to take the actual dead heart.

I wanted it, but was overruled by the highly curious medical establishment and their need for research grants.

Julia: When my son was 10, he wanted to take the neighbor's boa to Cub Scouts. There I was holding a 4' snake while the other den mother was clear across the yard.

If he'd taken a feather boa to Cub Scouts instead, it wouldn't have made your life any easier.

Serge: If you leave the state, will you sing "I left my heart in Colorado"?

Cindy: My dad had been in a minor car accident and had staples on the shallow cut on top of this bald head. Eldest wanted to take HIM to show-and-tell.

Alaena: Alas, most of them thought it was gross. Jasper and I thought it was cool.

Not just gross,' grandpa-gross.'

Elise: How many kids have a grandfather who had a heart transplant?

Janet: How many people know a heart transplant person at all?

Alaena: Perhaps I'll thaw out the bovine heart in my freezer and we can cross slice it like the picture for comparison.

Toni: So you're a jinx then?

Just walked a mile in 15:11, 4 mph. That's as fast as I ever walked it before.

Christine: You practicing your warm-up and cool downs?

Me: Sort of.

Maria: I can't go that fast even on a good day.

4/26/19
25 medical bills just came to our email at 12:30 in the flipping morning. I'll bet those are horrific.

Debbie: I was wondering about that...$200,000. I'm totally guessing here. I hope you have some type of health insurance!

Me: It'll be a lot more than that. Heart transplants are around a million bucks.

Closer to $2 million, so far. You could buy 1/40 of a pro athlete for that.

Me: Our insurance limits our annual out-of-pocket to $4000, thankfully.

And we're far past that. It's a joy to just go the pharmacy, get handed $8000 in rejection meds, and walk out without paying. Of course, I've been paying a monthly extortionate amount for decades.

Debbie: I originally put $400,000, but changed it not to stress you out. A million!!!!! ...unbelievable.

$400,000 turned out to be close to the negotiated price with the insurance company.

Ana: Yeah, I would say around a million. I dealt with complicated children heart transplant cases that can only be done in Boston, and those were 2 mil. You didn't stay much in the hospital and didn't need a lung to come with it or had other complications, so I would say somewhere a little over 1 mil.

Linda: FREE IN CANADA! Should be free in the States, as well, but...and no insurance required.

I should move there for that, and for the curling. But my tolerance for poutine is pretty low. It'd probably slay the new heart.

FYI: poutine...French fries and cheese curds, topped with brown gravy. A Quebec original. There's a theory that the name comes from Provencal French for 'bad stew.'

Veronica: That's what you get for leaving the hospital. They miss stealing your blood at all hours, so they're going for the second-best.

Maria: Glad you're on the mend, Terry. Wait awhile to look at those god-damned bills.

Me: I'm already on blood pressure meds because of the surgery and the other meds.

Cal: Thought about that...Well, since you are too young for Medicare, your insurance must have a cap, right? $6,000 or so?

Me: $4,000 a year, thank Odin.

Alaena: I thought you converted to Aztec? Thank Quetzalcoatl?

Quetzalcoatl ("feathered serpent"): the Aztec god of wind, air, and learning. Perfectly describes me. My students say that my teaching is all wind.

Me: Closing in on $1,000,000 already and the bills aren't all in yet.

Garalt: You may have to pay for Botox yourself.

Looks like the heart transplant bill is around $811,000 and rising.

Ana: That's some pretty good turn around on billing.

Me: They want to bill me quick in case the heart gets rejected.

If they don't get their $, they may send repo men around to our house with bone saws.

Julia: Think they would give you a refund if it did.

AE: Guess you'll be gettin' a second job — greeter at Walmart?

Jo: If you were in the UK, it would be free on the NHS.

Unless the Tories Brexit everything and dismantle it. Then you're back to prayer and leeches.

Maria: American healthcare — brought to you by a bunch of the greediest bastards in the world.

One insurance CEO makes $22 million a year. For doing what? I wouldn't pay that to somebody for curing cancer.

I mean, it's not like he plays a **sport***.*

Serge: Heart of gold?

Me: At less than a pound, that would be MUCH cheaper, actually.

About $1000 that way.

Mark: Good thing you have a new heart to take the shock.

The old one took a shock just fine.

CS: So, if you didn't have insurance, would you still get the procedure? And if so, then what? Bankruptcy?

Me: No insurance, no heart. Because you couldn't afford the meds to keep you going.

Alaena: It was very clear in the paperwork that your access to insurance and your ability to maintain $$ to pay for the ongoing medication etc. is highly figured into being listed on the transplant list in the first place.

CS: That's objectively evil.

Alaena: It is, but alas it's reality.

Bill: Do they charge by the beat?

That'd be $100 a minute, $6000 an hour, $144,000 a day, $52,560,000 a year.

Irritatingly, that would only be the annual income of the 17ᵗʰ richest pro athlete.

Tim: If a million of your friends each donate $1.00 this will be taken care of.

Just walked another 5K. Thought I was doing a leisurely stroll, but it was faster than the one I did Sunday. 17 minutes a mile. Conditioning improves without trying.

Picked up a 3-month supply of the two primary anti-rejection meds today. $25 co-pay per month. Cost without insurance: $4000. $1300 a month. $16,000 a year.

FYI, these are the GENERIC prices.

Marisa: That's insane.

You hear that word a lot with this transplant stuff.

Matthew: I suggest you hang on to that insurance.

(Meme) "I may not have the best body, but it holds all of my organs in place."

Me: Well, more or less.

It has help now. Stainless steel sternum wires. Haven't checked their TV reception yet.

4/27/19
Finally managed to get all of the adhesive off of my body from IV's and heart monitor patches. The hospital gave us some chemical swabs made just for that. Now all that's there are horrifying Frankenstein wounds.

Matthew: I STILL haven't been able to get all the adhesive off of my arms from my hospital stay. Which ended on March 3rd!

Me: The little wipes they gave us are made just for that. Work like a charm.

Matthew: What's in 'em? Soap? Rubbing alcohol? Nail polish remover? None have helped!

Me: Acetone, mostly.

Which also the term people have for my singing.

Victoria: Uni-solve. You can buy liquid or wipes like alcohol swabs.

Serge: It's 'FrankenSTEEN'!

David: Now go out and terrify the villagers!

Me: I already terrify them with my intellect, though this takes less social interaction.

Linda: Those aren't wounds they are badges!

We don't need no stinkin' badges!

From Mel Brooks' seminal work of postmodern American history, 'Blazing Saddles.' Lovingly ripped off from 'The Treasure of the Sierra Madre.'

The mandatory manscaping from the April 2 ablation (they ran catheters through both femoral arteries) is still jarring. #tmi #oversharing

Liana: You're upsetting my Victorian sensibilities.

As it grows back, I'll trim it into the hedge maze from 'The Shining' (film).

Or the topiary from 'The Shining' (book).

Fun fact: The Overlook Hotel from this novel is based on the creepy Stanley Hotel in Estes Park, Colorado, the town where I had my first Colorado teaching job. Stephen King lived in Boulder in the mid-1970's, visited that hotel, and was inspired to write the novel here.

My surgeon immediately after the heart transplant. (photo 52)

Me: Alternatively: **(photo 53)**

Serge: Blucher!

"My grandfather's work was…doodoo!" (yes, Mel Brooks actually has Oscar, Emmy, and Tony awards for quality writing)

4/28/19
Mom, brother, and sister flying in tomorrow for their first visit here from Illinois ever in the 21 years I've been in Colorado. For two of them, their first time on an airliner (mom's 80, sister's 58). And all I had to do to get this visit was have my heart ripped out.

Me: And Wednesday I'm making them drive me to my biopsy appointment in the big city. That'll show 'em.

Julie: That is evil. Traffic there is nuts!

Mandy: You make it sound like you got sacrificed to Quetzalcoatl.

Well, to United Health Care, Inc. anyway.

4/29/19
3 weeks ago I was just waking up from the transplant, that miserable breathing tube so far down my throat it was almost out of my ass. The waking up part was a mild surprise. I honestly didn't expect to, my luck not usually running in a positive direction.

Thankful that they chose not to remove it via my ass.

Maria: Dude, you had like half the Facebook rooting for you. It would have been a rotten thing to do not to wake up from that surgery.

Me: I would've been SO selfish.

Julia: Not only people who are Facebook friends of yours, but friends of friends of friends.

Maria: How is breathing these days? Is it getting any easier yet?

Me: Breathing's okay. I can walk a 5K without any problems. Can sleep on my side again. Turning over in bed doesn't hurt if I'm careful. Coughing and sneezing still suck.

Tim: It gets better every week.

Since I was born a month premature, hauled out with forceps on my skull, while mom was in a coma, I shouldn't be surprised at my current medical adventure.

Maria: Hey, I'm an 8-month preemie, too, as is my husband! We are survivors!

Janet, too. Good thing I'm not premature in every arena or she'd be more distraught than she already is.

Just another day in paradise. (photo 54)

Sharon: I take almost as many and I still have my original heart. Hmm…

Sharon, you know we love you, but...this is an intervention.

Maria: Colorful!

Me: The pretty blue and orange ones kill your immune system, but adorably.

4/30/19
I was reminded yesterday that even though you may be 61, bald, wrinkled, and infirm, your mom still thinks you're 7.

Veronica: Some of you is 19.

Thanks to the compromised immune system, I take Lysol wipes to restaurants, etc. and sterilize everything. So now I'm basically Adrian Monk. (photo 55)

From the award-winning TV show where a detective with psychological issues has germaphobia as one of his symptoms. His assistant had to follows him everywhere with a box of sterilizing wipes.

Me: Though I look more like Hector Elizondo than Tony Shaloub.

That's Hector on the left.

Maria: Naw, I love me some Hector, but there is no way he could rock an Elizabethan ruff with the same panache as you do.

Sharon: When are you going to write another book? Heart Xplant in Shakespearean?

I already look like Coriolanus, who was aptly named, because the character's an asshole.

Twice a day I take 4 big capsules in Denver Broncos colors. They literally keep me alive. Not sure how I feel about that. #ihatethebroncos,that'showIfeelaboutthat

Naturally, somebody who's into cycling, cricket, and curling has no interest in football whatsoever. The latter, especially, as the locals here all treat the Broncos like revealed religion. Every year we hope that they don't make the playoffs, so everybody on TV will shut up about them for a while.

Cerene: Old gods devour that which displeases them.

Me: The old gods are scared shitless of me.

To access the photos/videos/links:
www.terrykroenungink.com/246-2/

6) IT'S SINKO DE MAYO!

MAY 1-JUNE 30, 2019

This section gets us into the daily grind of recovery, after the April baby steps and frequent misery. I got into a routine with the meds, diet, and exercise. That routine was known as 'Jesus, Mary, and Joseph! Why is there no routine???' Meds would change as the team adjusted them to keep a balance of rejection stuff with all of the other prescriptions, diet would change because of the stomach issues, bathroom habits would change because of the intestinal issues on days when there were no stomach issues. The medication debacles with the insurance company and pharmacies tested my newly installed heart (and my Wellbutrin prescription). I'm happy to report that the ticker did not explode, and neither did my former temper tantrums. As of this writing in mid-July, I haven't turned purple, screamed, and broken things since well before the surgery (we aren't counting ordinary snippy fits at life's indignities). I feel like an addict who, similar to a naked monk, finally got rid of his habit. Keeps the wife and dog happier. It's bad enough that one of us here already walks around the house with tremors.

In May I continued the power walking, since that was the only real exercise I was allowed. Got up to doing 5-mile walks at about 4 miles per hour, which was as fast as I was doing with the old heart when it was healthy. In June the Mayo Clinic boffins informed us that my heart had not a whisper of amyloidosis in it, strangely enough, just sarcoidosis, and it only had a tiny fraction of actual muscle left. To this day no doctor can tell me why it was still beating, other than just to screw with them for a while longer.

To prevent dying if boredom, which would've been positively embarrassing after all of the decidedly non-boring stuff that returned me to the land of the living, we kept taking goofy transplant-adventure photos. Apart from that, I put this hunk of deathless prose together. Let's hope it's not the only deathless thing around here for a while. I'm not sure how generous my insurance company will be paying for a funeral, with all of the profit I've cost them.

5/1/19
Biopsy day. They won't let me eat after midnight. No water, either. Apparently, they're afraid I'll turn into a gremlin.

Too long to explain. Watch the 1984 move to get the joke. It's a heartwarming Christmas classic.

RaeAnne: I wonder if you realize what an inspirational person you are. You take situations that others could bemoan about and make them actually hysterical. I continue to pray for your healing and love your posts.

Mandy: I think he needs to write a book about this experience.

Me: Working on it. 40 pages of FB posts already transcribed.

Kate: Does Janis Joplin's "Piece of My Heart" get stuck in your head every time you do this procedure? Okay, now it will. You're welcome.

You are chaotic evil.

Veronica: They really like to keep you from eating.

SJ: Well, they don't want your fresh heart to fall out or anything.

Joe: And all this time I thought you were a Wookie! LOL

Adam: I read that as Gherkin.

Well, I was in quite a pickle until the transplant.

Liana: I've shared many of your posts with my husband due to his career running hospitals. He is flabbergasted at your progress, but mostly your sense of humor about it. We both applaud your courage (even if it was bravado) in facing this with as much levity as is possible with such a dire possible outcome. I imagine a jointly-written book with Janet would be cathartic for you both and a help for other patients and their partners going through similar crises. A thought.

Nice to know that I can flabbergast people for reasons other than my compulsive punning or autistic compulsions.

Me: It's in progress.

Alaena: Ohhhh, do I get to be in a book??

Me: We'll make sure the world knows about you contemplating running over a cyclist to score me a heart.

Rebecca: That is a very special daughter.

Alaena: Yay!! My neighbors will be horrified.

Note to anyone thinking about doing this: A) you really shouldn't, and B) try not to damage the bike. Those things are expensive.

Debbie: Couldn't agree more. Following him has been better than watching *Game of Thrones*! What he has gone through is unbelievable and taking those who wanted to support and be part of his journey has been a honour! Hell, I don't even know the guy and he now is my hero!!! I've talked about him to family and friends on all challenges he has faced and how he conquered them like it was nothing. They now ask me how Terry is doing...to say he hasn't touched and affected others is an understatement. I check him every day to make sure we're always on track.

Just found the pathology report in the old heart. It weighed 500 grams. Normal is 275-340. Ejection fraction was 20%. Should be no less than 55%. 80% of the heart muscle was gone, replaced by the sarcoid/amyloid.

Me: I lost over 10 lbs. in the hospital, but my heart got fat.

Alaena: Damn.

Me: How the hell can you be alive with only 20% of your heart muscle left???

Alaena: They should be asking you that.

Liana: My question is, "How did you manage all that walking and other exercising with so little heart muscle?"

My myocardial cells are few, but mighty.

And now they're literally on steroids.

Old dumb joke: Q: What do you get from sitting on cold concrete steps at the gym? A: Stairoids.

Lisa: You must have been getting around on sheer will power alone!

Julie: There's evidently a reason you need to be here.

Hopefully it's not just so I can finish this book. If so, I need to drag it the hell out.

Deborah: 70% is the highest number in heart function. So if you're running at 20% it's not as bad as it sounds. I only have 30% left of mine and I'm getting an implant defibrillator put in on the 15th.

Believe me, the cardiologists here sure acted like it was as bad as it sounds. They freaked.

Shae: EF should run between 50 to 70%. Anything below 50% is considered suspect and can lead to heart failure. Cardiomyopathies of various etiologies (causes or origins) cause low EFs, certain arrhythmias, valvular malfunctions, and damage from MIs. *(myocardial infarctions: heart attacks)* But interestingly, some people manage to function fine on very low EF's, while others suffer intense problems while EF's are still in marginal zones. Treatment all depends on the cause of course, but many times they can improve EF's significantly. In Terry's case, with those stats...it was amazing that he was alive, let alone standing.

Deborah: Thanks. I also have COPD and rheumatoid arthritis, so I barely get out of bed anymore!!

Shae: Oh my...I am so sorry. That is a wicked threesome to have. I am losing heart function due to an idiopathic arrhythmia...and I'm from a family with no heart issues of any kind of either side. The diagnosis was a blow. My EF is dropping 3 % a year and I'm losing my stamina as it declines. They think the damage was done by a simple virus I had years ago. In fact, the leading reason for heart transplantation these days are virus induced issues. But I doubt that would ever be in my cards. I don't have RA, but I have numerous autoimmune problems that make life difficult. I hope they can do something for you!

Pat: Tell you what fella, you must fancy your odds on the old Lottery now!

I figure I already won, so scoring twice would be a bit much to ask for.

Shannon: Holy crapola.

Garalt: Terry, most people talk about their I.Q. or golf handicap....just sayin'.

Believe me, an EF of 20 is a handicap.

Sarah: Hoo, hoo, look who knows so much? You were only mostly dead.

And there's our 'Princess Bride' allusion.

Suzann: Is the word miserable even in your vocabulary?

Jacqueline: Thank God they whipped it out before it just gave out!

That may be the first time a woman has said, "Thank God they whipped it out."

It's May Day and I'm lying on a hospital gurney. Time to lead the nurses in a rally for workers' rights while singing "The Internationale."

"We demand an end to forced stool-sample collection! Vive la Revolution!"

Liana: Do you have on a red gown?

Alas, no. It's the usual ugly-ass green. If I decide to run for it, I can hide in tall grass as the bloodhounds frantically scour the grounds for me, searchlights and sirens splitting the night air.

No sedation for the biopsy today, so I got to watch a TV with only one channel: my beating heart with a catheter in it, and my sawn sternum with wires holding it together. Hey, the screen was brighter than the Battle of Winterfell.

A 'Game of Thrones' allusion, because this ordeal seems nearly as long as the 10-year run of that show.

Eileen: Honey, midnight under a blanket was brighter than the Battle of Winterfell.

5/2/19
Waking up with a sore jugular vein a couple of days after watching a Vlad the Impaler documentary is a bit surreal.

Paul: Good job you decided to give that Wayne Bobbitt doc a miss, then.

Go ahead and Google that one, kids. Your collective wince will be epic.

And once again the pharmacy is refusing to give me the med order that the transplant office called in yesterday. Some insurance screw-up again. Waiting at the Safeway Starbucks for my team to fix it. Apparently, they're all in a staff meeting with their phones off. Off! Who does that???

Update: all fixed.

Eric: If it keeps happening, you should really think about buying stock in Starbucks.

Fun fact: Starbucks was originally going to be called Pequod's, after the ship in 'Moby Dick.' But they immediately realized that people were unlikely to enthusiastically embrace the idea of drinking anything from a cup with the 'pee' sound in its name.

Mary: It's like running a small country.

Since the biopsies are all clean, next week is my last weekly clinic visit. After that I'll only have to go to Denver every two weeks. Hopefully, they'll quickly go to monthlies.

Not that I don't love getting up before dawn for medical procedures and breakfast in a hospital cafeteria full of sick people…

It's pronounced Frahn-ken-STEEN! (photo 56)

Hang on, the 'Young Frankenstein' quotes are coming thick and fast!

Michele: What hump?

Liana: Walk this way...

Serge: Puttin' on the Ritz?

"Ah, sweet mystery of life, at last I've found youuuu!"

Cerene: You are so cool.

Valerie: I'm so sorry seeing your whole process. My husband passed away from a massive heart attack. If there was any chance, he would have suffered, but it was too late, they did everything they could to revive him. You are now my superhero. God bless you, now that you're 19 again.

Matthew: Hello, handsome!

Perry: Is that a zipper? For easy maintenance?

Velcro was too expensive.

Christine: This can't get any better!!

Linda: I have a zipper from above the point of my left shoulder to halfway down my upper arm. Staples out Monday. Still looking for a pair of those

Boris Karloff elevator shoes to complete the look. Glad you're feeling well enough to be goofy!

According to the geniuses at the Mayo Clinic, where my heart samples were sent, there is NO amyloidosis there, only sarcoidosis. False positive. That's actually the best possible outcome, because 5 mg of daily Prednisone keeps the sarcoid suppressed. Nothing but a liver transplant would likely keep amyloid from building up in the heart again.

Kelly: So you didn't have that disease? You don't have to worry about the new heart ? Or you still do?

Me: Doesn't look like it. I had a DIFFERENT fatal rare disease.

Kelly: So will this new one affect new heart?

Marion: This is really confusing. Please dumb it down for us, teach!

Alaena: Sarcoidosis is bad and fast, but treatable (assuming it's diagnosed in time). 5mg of Prednisone for life should keep it in check. Amyloid is bad, it's usually slow, and there is NO treatment. Likelihood of it coming back to affect the heart or another organ was significant and would require ongoing major medical.

Cindi: Wow — what are the chances?

Me: It's crazy rare either way.

Just like my genius.

Walked another 5K. 49:11, pace of 15:51/mile. Average pulse of 113. Did another mile in the morning, so that's 4 miles of fitness walking, plus the usual moving around. 15,000 steps. Pure ego. Hoping to get out of most of the cardiac rehab sessions that start next week.

Yeah, that turned out to a waste of time after the first week. I went into it in better shape than anybody else there. A few minutes of walking and cycling wouldn't improve me.

♫ "I'm too sexy for my scars…too sexy…" (photo 57)

Jon: Maybe consider getting that as a tattoo?

Me: Tattoos are verboten. Compromised immune system.

Roger: I'm not sure the newly installed zipper is much better

Me: It's fake. Just glued on temporarily.

Ana: Henna, too?

Me: Probably okay. Breaking the skin is the issue.

By popular demand…the zipper pull. (photos 58)

Alaena: You really should wear that to your appointment next week to get the staples out. Wear the bolts too…just 'cause.

Debbie: Oh, My God! Only you would do that! You have way too much time on your hands.

Janet: He can't work for 4 months. That's one-on-one time, 24/7 for 4 months. We need all the distractions we can get.

Janet soon began to re-evaluate how much fun me being retired and underfoot would be someday.

Debbie: Can we buy him a puzzle or something

Rebecca: I sent him adult coloring books, but he has not touched them.

*If they'd been actual **adult** coloring books, I'd have touched the hell out of them.*

Janet: He's not a puzzle person, either. And nothing crafty. He's got a bunch of books that need finishing or editing and he can work on his heart transplant opus, hopefully.

Rebecca: The coloring helps me with meltdowns. I tried.

Roger: Frankinterry.

5/3/19
Just read a medical journal estimating the prevalence of cardiac sarcoidosis at only 2 cases in every million people. That's about 640 people in a U.S. population of 320 million. #i'mspecial

Me: Jeez, can't I just sprain an ankle like everybody else?

Alaena: And how many of those end in transplant? (Not a lot, from my guess when I was checking up on you).

Liana: Time to buy a lottery ticket.

Shae: Like my cardiologist says...it's not necessarily a good thing to be considered special when it comes to medical issues. Ah, well...

Could be worse. They could be holding a last-ditch telethon for me.

Or I could be on the cover if a supermarket tabloid: "His brave last days."

Just saw my local cardiologist, Dr. Carlyle, to keep her in the loop. If she hadn't ID'd my problem in February, I wouldn't be here right now. She was verklempt at my survival and progress. She'd followed all of my procedures on her computer. So happy, she literally almost cried.

Who says doctors are emotionless cure-machines?

I gave her a copy of this book later. Pretty sure that DID make her cry, and not with joy.

Nancy: She is a keeper.

This is true.

The Prednisone is building up in my system. Hands are shaking to the point of having trouble getting toothpaste onto the brush. I survived heart failure only to get Parkinson's symptoms.

Right now I'm on nearly half the original dose and my handwriting still looks like a drunken toddler's in a bouncy castle. Because tacrolimus causes tremors, too.

Me: Given the alternative, it's still a good tradeoff.

Alaena: After the 20mg, the steady 5mg should be a piece of cake. No playing with the good china in the meantime.

Ali: Didn't know it did that, and I know or have known a number of people who take it for sarcoidosis. Check whether you're taking too much.

Me: It's a big dose because it's for immunosuppression.

Ali: Do you mean they're using it as an anti-rejection as well as to treat the sarcoidosis?

Me: Temporarily, yes. They taper it off later.

Dave: Prednisone sucks giant donkey balls. I'm sorry, man.

Hey, donkeys need love, too (though teabagging may be a bridge too far).

Jeanne: How long do you have to stay on the Prednisone? I was on 40mg a day for several months and I didn't enjoy it. It's a miracle and a nightmare at the same time.

Me: 20 mg for a few months, then they taper to 5 mg forever for the sarcoid.

Can't imagine being on twice my dose. Holy hell...

Tim: I missed this. 5 mg is much easier to deal with. I'm down to 7.5 now.

Sharon: I have tremors, too. I guess there is a drug for it, but it causes arrhythmia problems and I have Long QT Syndrome. Not worth dying over.

That condition affects the repolarization of the heart after a beat. You can fall over dead with no warning from it.

Not to be confused with Long Cuticle Syndrome, which is an occupational hazard in nail salons.

Deena: Gah! I felt like a zombie after a 5-day infusion for MS. A literal zombie. Hoping this is only temporary for you and that once your down to maintenance level, you'll be back to steady.

Tim: The tacrolimus will do that as well.

Just freaked out my entire school by strolling in unannounced.

Not hyperbole. Thought I was going to have to defibrillate the office ladies.

Me: And now I'm stuck in the parking lot until the students' cars get out of my way.

Alaena: Should have timed that better.

Barbara: I know they were very surprised, but awfully glad to see you.

Serge: Did you have the neck bolts on?

They were rentals. Had to return them to get my deposit back.

Kelly: Were they happy to see you?

Either that or there were pickles in pockets.

Me: Looked like it.

Cruz: We were.

Cruz must be telling the truth. He already graduated and I have no leverage on him now.

Marisa: Anyone check if you were a white walker?

SO white. You have no idea. Janet had my DNA checked. Almost 100% Scandinavian, English, Scottish, Irish, German. I'm a phosphorescent walker.

When I showed photos of my dead heart at school, they all shouted "Oh, my freaking God!" Interestingly, the doctors all had exactly the same reaction.

Julie: This could make one of those kids be a doctor someday.

5/4/19
The fun and joy of being literally 1000% more susceptible to skin cancer. Ugly large-brimmed hat and long-sleeved shirt when it's pushing 80 degrees. Clothes are SPF 50. (photo 59)

I know it's entirely too sexy, but I just can't turn it off.

Me: At least I don't have to spray sunblock on my arms this way.

Cynthia: You are also 1000% untethered from machines measuring your various body functions and how soon they might give out. Be thankful, young man, for how far you've come in a month.

Julie: I guess you told him.

AE: Gloves — where are your gloves?

I lost them challenging a couple of asshats to duels.

Me: Sunblock.

AE: That's no fun! Have you tried the ole beekeeper's attire???

Stephany: You look lovely!

Russell: See, this is me all the time. I burn like a bastard. I have nicer hats, though. I mean... Damn!

Sheila: I think you look dashing.

Yeah, dashing through the sun to get to the shade.

Alaena: It'd look cute with a vest over it.

Jess: Hazmat suit?

Melisse: When my city (Casper, WY) was flooded with astronomers for the eclipse, we drove through town to see all the excitement. A whole group of astronomers set up in a huge parking lot. They all wore Outback/Australian bush hats and looked cool!

And they all had third-degree burns on one side of their faces.

Cerene: Tie-dye that shirt, you have no hippy showing.

Amber: But you could wear a wide-brimmed pirate hat and a pirate shirt every day and say it's for SPF!

Me: I like how you think.

John: All depends what the odds of catching it in the first place are. If they started at 1 in a billion, you'd be down to 1 in 100,000.

According to the wife, this new heart absolutely did NOT improve my social skills.

Ali: Surely you're not supposed to be doing that yet...ah, sorry, middle of the night here.

Don't call me Shirley.

Jim: What a disappointment!!!!!!

Jeanne: You're a moody teenager again!

Eileen: Well, it is only 19 years old.

Me: Some of y'all are **really** misconstruing what I mean by social skills.

But thanks for the romantic vote of confidence.

Maria: No, you'd need a brain transplant for that.

2-mile walk, 31:25. A 15:40 pace, almost 4 mph. Average pulse 114.

5/5/19
**Transplant was 4 weeks ago tonight. Coughing is starting to hurt a
LITTLE bit less. It still hurts like Hell, just not the 9th circle of it.**

Not Dante's 'Inferno.' More like 'Disco Inferno.'

*This reminds me that my tragic fate was that **all** of my middle school/high school/college
years were in the 1970's.*

It's Sinko de Mayo! (photo 60)

Maria: <groan>

Matthew: You were brought back from the brink of death...for this?

Absolutely. Your agony makes mine seem less.

Matthew D.: They took you apart to put in a whole new ticker, and you're
telling me they couldn't have done a sense of humour transplant, too?

Me: Apparently, I'm incurable.

They couldn't find a weird-enough donor for that.

I just found this amusing. (photo 61)

Andrea: In German, 'gift' means poison.

And in France, you can be poisoned by a gift of bad poisson.

Richard: Hey, my birthday's coming up, maybe get me some opioids while you're there?

Sorry, they say they're fresh out. There's a big rock festival in town.

5/6/19
5K walk, 16:30/mile. Tomorrow's one-month post-transplant. I jogged 10 steps as an experiment. Don't rat on me to the doctors. Well, I call it jogging. Probably couldn't have slid a sheet of paper under my heels. More like sad race-walking.

Me: Nothing hurt, nothing collapsed or exploded, no stroke. That might happen to my coordinator if she finds out, though.

Turned out she didn't care.

Dave: Yeah. Don't…do…that. Walking makes a lot of sense. Running with your parts flopping out after the staples tear, really not a good look for your neighborhood.

*My parts flopping out wouldn't be a good look for **any** neighborhood.*

Had to drive the car on Friday, since Janet's half-blind from her new meds. Another thing not to mention to my Transplant Team.

(Janet) There were varying opinions from different doctors on how long before Terry could drive. To hire a driver for a one-way trip to the hospital cost $100, so we are taking our chances.

Rebecca: I would yell at you, but it would not do any good.

Jess: REBEL!

I can't live by your rules!

Barbara: I hear no evil, see no evil.

Final (hopefully) weekly heart biopsy tomorrow. If everything's good on the rejection front, it goes to every 2 weeks for a while, then monthly. My abused jugular vein will thank them.

I looked like a heroin addict who ran out if usable veins elsewhere.

The 50 staples in my chest come out tomorrow. Woo-hoo!

Cindi: I think you should wear the zipper pull to your appointment.

Matthew: Not to mention the neck bolts. And brush up on "Puttin' on the Ritz."

> *"Come with me and we'll attend their jubilee*
> *And see them spend their last two bits*
> *Puttin' on the Ritz."*

Without insurance, I'd already be down to my last two bits, to pay for replacing my bits.

Liana: That'll be fun. Suggestion: count down, not up.

Chris: How will you celebrate? I know! You could go to Staples.

*It **would** help me achieve...closure.*

It's Nurses' Week. Teacher Appreciation Week, too.

Maria: So, what you are saying, it's superheroes' week?

"What's that in the sky? It's a bird! It's a plane! No, it's an Overworked/Underpaid Public Servant!"

Getting a bone density scan tomorrow morning, checking for osteoporosis from the meds. The transplant has turned me into an old lady.

Maria: You don't need bones for 5-10 years? What will you do with them? Do you keep them in a closet under the stairs?

♫ *"Dem bones, dem bones, dem dry bones…"*

Me: It was all I could do to not say to the radiologist, "Look at the bones!" in a John Cleese voice.

I'm betting that wouldn't have been the first time. I didn't want to be the one who sent the tech into a homicidal rage from it.

Bren: That's for them to compare with in the future…because those drugs you're taking are going to interfere with bone density.

Me: I'm on wagonloads of calcium/vitamin D, Fosomax, and dietary calcium for that.

BTW, Fosomax sucks (even my doctors say so). You take it once a week to prevent osteoporosis and it wrecks your stomach with fires of Hades in return. They switched me to Boniva (who comes up with these names?) and it was much better.

5/7/19
At the hospital again for the last weekly biopsy, etc. All of the appointments have called us in early, which never happens. The blood draw barely hurt and the bone scan only required taking off my belt. Everything's so ahead of schedule that now we have 45 minutes to kill waiting for the Transplant Team clinic meeting. Biopsy's immediately after that, then a 2 1/2 hour wait to get the staples removed. Hoping to save some of the staples to stick in a scrapbook or art installation or whatnot.

Janet's working on that art piece as we speak. Hilariously, she's having trouble getting the staples to stick to the board.

Ali: You could maybe arrange the staples on pics of sections of your old heart, maybe holding the sections together, or forming a word or symbol. Ask to keep them all.

Mark: Put them on a ring or necklace.

Genital piercings.

Looks like I have personalized hospital socks. (photo 62)

Julie: What color are they?

Me: Brown. So they made me walk to the OR.

Julie: You're too well for the Big Bird socks.

I still want green Oscar the Grouch socks.

My biopsy lab and the whacky nurses. (photos 63, 64)

It's usually the same group whenever I'm there. They're goofy enough that I bet they're a hoot at Anschutz Cardiac Karaoke Night.

Blood drawn (levels are perfect), bone scan done, clinic done (took me off of the stomach-wrecking Fosomax), biopsy done (actual doctor procedure took maybe ten minutes; heart skipped beats when the catheter went into the right atrium—that's normal). Now waiting another hour to get the staples yanked (if they walk in with one of those terrifying claws we pull staples with at school, I'm out.

Maria: Could be even more interesting if they show up with a magnet.

Jim: I think they contract that work out to Magneto.

The nurse just tried to find a pulse in my right wrist and failed. That's the wrist that turned black from bruising. Vessels are still a mess.

Samantha: Nurses can never find my pulse in my wrist for some reason. I always joke that I must be dead.

"I'm sorry, we must drive a wooden stake through you. It's best for community safety."

Serge: Cue in the "I'm not dead yet" scene from *Holy Grail.*

"I feel happy! I feel happy!" (that's why Happy took out a restraining order on me)

The nurse just came into the waiting room and called for 'Mrs. Brown.' It took all of my willpower to not sing ♫ "You've got a lovely daughter."'

Peter: Oh, go ahead and sing next time.

No, my singing is a prosecutable crime against humanity.

Wanda: Herman and the Hermits.

Bonnie: I wish you were my patient. We would get along swimmingly.

Virginia: I worked for eye doctors for a while, and I had to call a patient whose surname was Duck. I'm not kidding. I could not do it. Every time I started laughing. "Mr. Duck?"

Please tell me his first name was Don.

Me: I had an Army dentist named Toothaker.

Toni: My dentist as a child was Dr. Bone. Later, my doctor's surname was Dick, which had my little boys suggesting what his first name might be. Quite entertaining.

I swear to Odin, I knew a guy in my hometown in Illinois named Les Dick.

Scott: In my life, I have encountered: An eye surgeon named Dr. Fry. Yes, he had the Fry Eye Clinic; a police reporter named Shields; a traffic engineer named Street. This is how I learned the word "aptonym."

Cindi: I had a client named Olive Pitts, and she married into the name! Lol

And once again the Cardio-Thoracic Surgery unit has wasted an hour of my time (so far) because they seem to think that appointment times are merely suggestions.

Janet: Threaten them with a trip over to the Cardiac Clinic to let them pull them out. This is ridiculous.

If I take their fee away, they may come to my house and re-install the old heart.

Jim: They're more like guidelines, really...

Staples out. Yes, we kept them. Transplant surgeon thought the zipper pull photo was a hoot.

Barbara: I bet it hurt, though, when they took the staples out.

Me: Not really.

Mildly disappointing. Something I couldn't complain about.

Rebecca: Let the scratching begin.

Looks even more Frankensteiny with the staples out. (photo 65)

Treva: Looks like an interesting tattoo.

Maria: Ow.

Me: Didn't hurt, actually (the staple removal, anyway).

Cindy: Great healing!!!

Sharon: You look fantastic, for what you have been through.

Barbara: That will fade with time. I had 31 staples from sternum to belly button, and you can hardly see the scars anymore. I'm so happy for you!

Debbie: I'm waiting for you to tell us you acted this whole play out...and the joke's on us. I can't believe you went through all of this with flying colors. Mind-blowing, really. I'm beginning to wonder if you're one of us...I watch way too much TV.

*Cue the creepy "One of us!" chant from the creepy 1932 movie 'Freaks.' **(link #6)***

You got me. This whole time I've been sipping margaritas in Tahiti and inventing fake FB posts.

SF: It's Fronken-steeny!

Sheila: I think it's rather neat. I'd make it a feature in my couture.

Janus: You are now an official member of the zipper club!

Giselle: There are now products which will reduce scarring that you can buy from the pharmacist.

Tim: They used glue on mine. The scar actually healed nicely.

Alessandro: Chicks dig scars.

Janet actually thinks it's cool, which is way out of character.

5/8/19
Staples, glue, constant hand sanitizing, writing reports, going to meetings...surgeons are just elementary school teachers with knives.

Maria: ...and hacksaws.

Me: Circular saw, in my case.

Maria: Oh, pardon me, Mr. Sophisticated.

They got a bit over-eager on the biopsy yesterday. My jugular and sternomastoid muscle ache like hell. Hard to swallow. Or maybe 4 biopsies in 3 weeks, plus a solid week of having a port in the same spot before that, is more than my poor neck can handle.

Rebecca: Did you call your doctors? I have a feeling I know the answer.

Me: No swelling, bleeding, or discoloration. I'm keeping a watch on it.

Rebecca: I knew that was your answer.

Me: Getting better already. Neener-neener.

Apparently, the staples were supporting my poor torso more than you'd think. Now moving is more achy than before. Plus, the deep bruising is still increasing and hurting. But the doctors say those ugly green bruises are a good sign of healing, so...

Well, of course they'd say that. "Look at those big beautiful green suckers, you lucky bastard..."

Stephany: So maybe the doctors knew what they were talking about when they said rest? And maybe someone has been overdoing the exercise? Just a little?

Cal: 19-year-old's spirit? Great film material with humor, bringing the boomer with millennial.

Stephany: It's not the 19-year-old. It's the 61-year-old who still wants to pretend he's 19. I do like the film idea.

I notice that 19 and 61 are basically the same number upside-down and reversed... like my life.

Janet: A few rainy days to relax on the couch might be a good thing. Sleep helps, too, and two days of early wake-up requires some rest.

Rebecca: Listen to your wife.

If I start doing that after all this time, it may give her a heart attack, and we know how much those cost.

Blah-blah-blah...'common sense'...blah-blah-blah...

I count 11 slices and punctures on my corpus. 12 inches of incisions. Jack the Ripper's victims looked better. But at least I have the same number of organs that I started with, so that's a plus.

Couldn't say that about the appendectomy, though a gangrenous one really isn't a keeper. Looked like a zombie penis (I imagine).

Really didn't think I'd be typing 'zombie penis' in a heart transplant memoir. But then, I ever thought I'd be typing a heart transplant memoir, either.

Rebecca: Although you do have a pre-owned part.
At least it's under warranty. 5 years or 50 million beats, with free tune-ups.

It occurs to me that my heart isn't old enough to drink. #goaheadandcardme

Russell: Come to the U.K. You'll be fine.

Karen: It is in Canada!

Rebecca: You can't buy cigarettes, either.

Matthew: #goaheadandcardiome

I'll just slap a moustache on it and have it beat in a deep voice.

4th biopsy totally negative for rejection. Don't have to do it again for 2 weeks.

Me: Maybe the neck will be all in one piece by then.

Because having to go in through a rectal vein would be a major pain in the…well, you know.

The new Vogmask arrived. Now I can venture out into germier environments, protected by cartoon doggies. I look like the lamest villain in a *GI Joe* movie. (photo 66)

Jeff: Aren't you in the next Marvel movie trailer?

Me: I'm Captain Doofus.

Mark: It's Bane!

I still have a vein section in each arm that feels and looks like a solid leather tube. Disconcerting. I pointed this out at the hospital yesterday and they said not to worry, it's just the vessels complaining about too damned many IV's. It'll go away on its own eventually. In the meantime, it looks like I'm smuggling drug packets subcutaneously.

Mark: Keep an eye on it in years ahead, Terry. My mother's veins got so bad from the same type of over-use that they packed up and no-one could get blood from them. Needed to have a portacath implanted for access in her chest with a line to her heart. Not to scare you, just worth watching if they're going to continue with lots of blood-taking.

Me: Won't have arm IV's again unless something goes very sideways.

Fingers crossed, knocking in wood, throwing salt over the proper shoulder…

Yeah, I'm insane. 5K run July 21, organ donor benefit in Denver. 105 days post-transplant. #needagoal

Me: They have a walking division, if I can't jog a 5K by then.

Which is mostly what happened, thanks to nagging little leg injuries that kept me from training.

Alaena: That's doable. And it's not like you have to "race."

5/9/19
About to drive through a snowstorm, in the second week of freaking May, to do my first cardiac rehab session at the hospital. They want me to go 3 days a week, which I'm guessing will be a colossal waste of my time at my current level of conditioning. The big thing on Day 1 is to walk for 6 minutes. I can do 10 times that without breaking a sweat. Just save the slot for somebody who really needs it.

Treva: But the snowstorm drive should be a good cardio test.

A test of my stroke risk, at least.

Cal: I was thinking the same. I had a B&N book signing and drove w/dog thru snowstorm...heart workout, for sure. Great adventure. Not.
Bill: I went to cardio rehab two separate times. They'll hook you up to live monitors to see how your new ticker is working in its new host. We had a (very) few patients end up in the ER once they pressed too hard. I found it fun and I really needed the regular exercise.

It's a bit counterintuitive that after they puncture your jugular vein with a ginormous needle and run 3 catheters into your beating heart, they just slap a band-aid on it and shove you out the door. #notevenjoking

Maria: Well, they don't want you becoming a sissy.

At least they don't pour gunpowder in and set it off. Or use a branding iron.

The full glorious spectacle of cardiac rehab. As usual, they were agog at my fitness. They said I'm not their typical customer. (photo 67)

Alaena: So, a REALLY expensive gym membership.

Me: Only cost a million bucks plus.

Ali: It looks like a torture chamber.

A torture chamber of boredom.

Just ordered this. Because of course I did. (photo 68)

Nothing calms you down like squeezing an anatomically-correct heart.
Except doing it to the hearts if your enemies and hearing the lamentation of their women.

*Allusion to 1982's 'Conan the Barbarian." But I don't have to tell **you** that.*

*The villain, James Earl Jones, as he's about to crucify Arnold Swarzenegger: "Look at the strength in your body, the desire in your **heart**, I gave you this!" Pretty sure my cardiologist said the same thing to me, as I lay crucified by IV lines and urinary catheters.*

5/10/19
Truth. (photo 69)

I'm 61 and I'm the youth movement at cardiac rehab.
One of the guys is older than God and has been going to this rehab for TWENTY years.

Laura: When I go to my cardiologist, I'm always the youngest — when I was still seeing a pediatric cardiologist, I was the oldest!

David: I'd go for 20 years if my insurance would cover it!

Me: He's 96 (!)

The rehab specialist apologized for boring me with her required, but lame, starter exercises on Day 1 today. The other 3 guys in the class are all textbook heart attack body types. Barrel-shaped. Don't know how long they've been doing rehab, but their hearts aren't going to do well if they don't change that.

Barbara: Some of the barrel shape may also be due to COPD, so if they smoke, they gotta quit.

5/11/19
5-mile walk in 1:21:17. 16:15/mile. Average pulse 112. 11,500 steps before noon.

Serge: Cue in the opening narration from *The Six Million Dollar Man.*

Me: Not planning to make that a daily habit quite yet, though.

Good thing we met our out-of-pocket max on the medical bills. 30 days of my valganciclovir (for **CMV** virus prevention) at retail price is **$20,000 a year**. At those prices, it ought to bestow literal immortality.

I need to name the new heart. Leaning towards Archie McThump-Thump.

Rebecca: Hearty McHeartface.

Mike: I'd go more along the lines of Beatachest Cumbervalve.

Mark: Johann Gambolputtydevon.

Mark: Spiny Norman. "Dinnesdale!"

Yeah, you'd expect Mark to go with the obscure Python reference.
In college in the 70's, I adapted a bunch of Monty Python skits into a 1-act play called "A Rather Silly Way for 5 Grown Men to Behave." The cast was 4 men and a woman. Mark was one of those 5. Extra points for guessing which.

I sent the script to the Pythons for permission to perform it as at theatre class project. Not only did they say yes, they edited the script and returned it on Terry Gilliam letterhead. #classy

Chris: T. Rands Plant.

Me: Cardio-B.

Donna: This!!!!

Jenn: THIS WINS!

Taylor: Ding-ding-ding! We have a winner!

Maria: Nebuchadnezzar.
Julie: Robert Bruce.

Johnnie: Donald Thump.

You're dead to me, Johnnie.

Ted: Doctor Beat.

Scott: Maybe you should name after the person who gave it to you.

Me: Unknown. May never be known.

Cindi: They don't usually let recipients know who gave them the parts.

Linda: Thumper!

Caroline: Archie Mountbeaten-Windsor.

5/12/19
Well, this headline explains why my 'generic' immunosuppressive drugs are still insanely expensive.

"The level of corporate greed alleged in this multistate lawsuit is heartless and unconscionable." (generic drug manufacturers caught colluding with one another to fix prices) (link #7)

How many damned yachts and houses can you use???

Exactly 5 weeks ago this hour I was on an operating table, chest open like a basement trap door, getting parts swapped out. It's all good, but it'll never stop being weird, bizarre, and surreal.

It's been several months as of this writing and that hasn't changed.

Then again, Janet says I've always been weird, bizarre, and surreal, so…

Tina: You've done great. It would be strange to have another's heart beating inside. It would take a while for me to absorb this miracle!

Debbie: This is probably one of the craziest questions anyone has asked….but do you feel different? You were always funny….so that hasn't changed. Enquiring minds want to know.

Me: Med side effects aren't bad, actually, but the heart is slower to react to movement, so getting up from the couch, I can feel sluggish or even briefly dizzy. But the heart is a Ferrari engine and once I get moving, I feel better than with the old one.

Maria: We wouldn't want you any other way. Glad Cerberus is taking good care of you.

Peter: But it'll never stop being weird, bizarre, and surreal. I believe it. I'm still confounded by the fact that this is now considered normal medicine in 2019.

Me: The doctors talk about it like it's fixing a sprained ankle.

If your ankle's made out of gold and diamonds.

Peter: Good Lord.

A new heart and 20 mg of daily Prednisone seems a long way to go to get clear skin.

5/13/19
At school for the past 90 minutes, getting the tech guy to fix my computer password issues, so I could finish my evaluation paperwork. He said it was so exotic, he hadn't done it in 5 years. Computer, heart...I have weird issues to fix no matter what I do.

Marisa: I'm fairly shocked you're at the school at all. What aren't there only like 3 days left?

Me: Needed to be on the school network to fix the computer. Not actually working until fall.

Maria: Does your computer need a transplant, too?

Me: A password transplant. All fixed.

An Apple laptop. Who's surprised?

Cardiac rehab: trying to be excited about running and biking to nowhere.

Maria: Why can't they just let you do it outside and record yourself?

Because they don't get paid that way, I'm figuring.

Julie: This is why I don't do gyms. You walk to nowhere. You bike to nowhere. You pick up heavy things and put them down for no reason at all. If I want to lift heavy things, I'll vacuum under the sofa.

Bearing the burden of my genius alone is quite the workout.

5/14/19
The wife seems strangely enamored of my 9-inch incision. "It's the scar. Chicks dig the scar."

Callback to one of the Batman movies.

Cheri: It's true. Chicks dig scars. It's a thing.

Tina: Maybe, if you play your cards right, she'll kiss each staple scar ?!?!?!?

Toni: You're G.I. Joe now, with lifelike scar.

"Now with real orthotopic allograft action!"

Orthotopic means 'a tissue transplant grafted into its normal place in the body.' An allograft is 'a tissue graft from a donor of the same species as the recipient, but not genetically identical.' In other words, the tissue isn't from you, like a skin graft, but from someone else.

43 pages, 12,000 words (and counting), of snarky heart transplant FB posts transcribed for the eventual book about all of this.

Because all of America is waiting in breathless anticipation.

5/15/19
Jogged 30 steps today without incident (don't tell the Transplant Team; they get salty at having their rules bent). Well, I call it a jog, but it was with our basset hound, so exceedingly impressive it was not.

Just did 50 more jog steps at 6 pm. Didn't warm up at all and Archie McThump-Thump let me know that he needs a little warning for that sort of thing.

"Dude, I was takin' a nap. WTF???"

Maria: I am sure you left many little old ladies and pregnant dogs in the dust behind you.

Me: Uh...not so much.

I didn't exactly rip the leaves from trees as I blazed past.

Ali: Presumably Archie is plumbed in, the joints still settling, but not fully wired into the mains/motherboard/brain. Wondering if some of the tedious rehab encourages new connections.

Me: The vagus nerve has to be cut to put a new heart in, so there's now no direct electrical connection to the brain to regulate heart response. That means longer warm-up to chemically alert the brain to raise the bpm for exertion.

Ali: This is what I guessed. Can it regrow?

Me: Sometimes. Takes 5-10 years if it does.

Not holding my breath on that one.

My new anatomically correct (more or less) squeezy stress ball. It's really disturbing when you squeeze it in a natural heart rhythm and make it expand and contract. (photo 70)

Creeps my students out.

Rebecca: At least you will be entertained for a few hours.

Julie: We want a vid of this.

It's on FB now. I can deny thee nothing, m'lady. (it got the predictable reaction)

Released from the hospital a month ago today. Everything's ticking along nicely, so to speak.

Me: At the risk of way too much information, **EVERYTHING'S** now working at the 19-year-old level.

Me: That'll help sell the book when it comes out.

Me: #nobluepill

Galen: EVERYthing?!?!?! OMG!

Me: Hey, I only report the news.

Cindi: I'm sure Janet Moongoddess loves that! I hear musical strains from *Young Frankenstein* emanating from your home..."Oh sweet mystery of life, at last I've found you!"

Donna: Visual is frightening.

Julie: My mind has too many options for a pithy retort here.

Sad to report, an eggplant emoji is actual size.

5/16/19
Watched a Peter Cushing Frankenstein flick from the 1960's yesterday. Hollywood has a VERY incorrect idea of how quick and easy it is to remove a human heart. *Last of the Mohicans* and every Aztec movie make the same mistake. Apparently, the sternum and ribs don't exist and it only takes a couple of snips to yank the thing out.

Liana: I suspect they are not awfully concerned with saving the arteries and veins for attachment of a new one, however.

They should be. You have to match all that stuff precisely when you install it into your soulless monster.

Serge: There's a scene in *Fantastic Voyage* that now makes me think of you. *Hopefully not the one where Donald Pleasance gets absorbed by white blood cells.*

Sitting on the couch with a pulse of 82. Which means that when I stand up, I'll have to hold onto the wall for a bit to let Archie catch up, because that bpm is actually my fall-asleep rate now.

5/18/19

Off to the Colorado Book Awards again. Last time (2017) was right before I got the pacemaker, and the anthology that I had a story in won the award. I have another story in a new version of the same anthology. If we win again, we'll know that my brushes with cardiac mortality are the key. FYI, I am **NOT** going through that again for the next one. #evenIhavelimits

Update: we didn't win, which got me out of having to accept the award for the absent editors and give a 3-minute reading. Now I can finish this beer.

(Mark Stevens) Yes, the one and only Terry Kroenung and his wife Janet at the Colorado Book Awards event tonight — Terry is just six weeks out after a heart transplant and looking like a million bucks! Terry was ready to read from the *False Faces* RMFW anthology, but "we" did not win. (photo 71)

Everybody keeps commenting on my wonderful color since the heart transplant. I don't see it myself, but I must've been as gray as a Scottish winter sky. #19yearoldheartimprovesthecirculation

Julie: How is your energy level?

Me: Fine so far.

Julie: Wow. Better looking and more energy already?! It can only go up from here.

Alaena: If you go back through the pictures, you were looking a bit splotchy for the last 6 months or so. Not really gray until the hospital, I think.
So by then I had Gray Anatomy?

5/19/19
6-weekaversary of the heart transplant. Hardly hurts the sternum to cough now, though the pacemaker removal site is still bruised and aching. At least that's improving, too.

Did another 50-step jog today. Archie McThump-Thump had no complaints. If he had, I guess I wouldn't be posting this.

5/20/19
6 weeks ago I had just awakened from the heart transplant with that wretched breathing tube in. Wasn't impressed with the actual breathing it was providing. Felt like a hostile alien symbiote, which is ironic considering that they'd just spent 7 hours implanting an actual symbiote.

Serge: Planning to work with Benjamin Sisko?

Adam: Change your name to Kroenung Dax.

Yes, dear reader, now you have to be up on 'Star Trek: Deep Space 9', too.

Spent the last couple of hours copying selected comments on my cardiac FB posts into the book document.

Maria: It shall be a volume to rival *War and Peace*.

Me: In how much it annoys readers, yes.

Me: I CAN guarantee that it'll be funnier than *War and Peace.*

5/21/19
Just picked up my doctor's note to get me out of potential jury duty in June. Being stuck with 11 germy strangers in very close quarters is not what my immunosuppressed self should be doing right now. Plus, the court's in Greeley. Hard pass on that.

Greeley: Full of cows, as far away as Denver, and precisely 1/10 as interesting.

Toni: Thanks for the reminder. I've been called to jury duty on my birthday. Over an hour away. Must admit you have a better excuse.

Not too late to make that happen. Bespoke cardiac transplantation is all the rage with the hipsters now.

(online article) "Why Lack of Sleep is Bad for Your Heart." (link # 8)

Oh, the irony, considering the utter lack of sleep I got in the hospital...in the HEART unit.

5/22/19
At the medical center again for another heart biopsy. 2 hours of nasty medication-induced reflux. This sucks. Feels like the heart attack they went to great trouble and expense to prevent.

Same thing happened the day of the next biopsy. Looks like it's not the meds, it's the medics. So I guess I'll just stay home and gauge my rejection status with a Ouija board.

Waiting to be hauled to the Catheter Lab for the latest biopsy. They let somebody with a heart attack jump the line. The nerve of some people.

Update: nearly 90 minutes past the appointment time and still waiting. About to lose my sense of humor.

Yeah, the nerve of some people. Probably the vagus nerve, in this case.

(Janet) It's certainly no fun sitting for up to eight hours in hospital waiting rooms surrounded by coughing, wheezing people, with the constant dings of phone updates and old ladies carrying on conversations on phones that don't need high-level decibels to work.

Beth: I believe you went ahead of a few people 6 weeks ago!!

Me: Most likely.

I was that guy on the highway when traffic narrows to one lane who races up to the front to jam himself in and doesn't even do that little 'apology wave.'

When they get you onto the biopsy table, they ask you what music you want them to play. Being the smartass that I am, I said, "Total Eclipse of the Heart." 60 seconds later, and I am NOT joking, it was coming out of the speakers. #trainedprofessionals

Literally total recall.

Randall: They must have Alexa. I scoffed at my son's when I asked it to play *Rhapsody on a Theme of Paginini*, and I'll be danged but a half hour later — on it comes! Actually, I find that sort of creepy. Visions of someone named Alexa running through an office asking everyone if they knew what that was! Glad you were able to get your tunes!

A work for piano and orchestra, written/performed by Sergei Rachmaninoff in the 1930's. Premiered in Baltimore, of all places. The most famous work associated with the capital of Maryland, except for that noted orchestral classic, 'Hairspray, the Musical.' Conducted by Leopold Stokowski, later husband of Gloria Vanderbilt and previously the conductor of 'Fantasia', favorite flick of stoners everywhere.

Niccolò Paganini was the first 'rock star.' His spectacular violin-playing, full of not merely gobsmacking technical perfection but showy tricks, movements, hair, and clothes, was so beyond what anyone else could do in the early 19th century that the Catholic Church accused him of having made a deal with the devil (indirectly, this is the inspiration for Charlie Daniels' 'The Devil Went Down to Georgia.'). He was so good that when he borrowed a priceless Guarneri violin, after hearing what Paganini could do with it, the stupefied owner refused to take it back.

Maria: This totally has to go into your book.

Me: All of this is going into the book.

And here it is. How prescient of her.

Andrea: Next time: "Unchain My Heart."

Chris: "My Heart Will Go On."

Julie: I think you need to have a playlist for these times.

Fiona: Can I suggest 'Achy breaky heart' as your next request?

My biopsy doctor looked like she was 14 years old and sang along with Sting and "Roxanne" while running probes into my jugular vein.

> ♫ *"Doctorrrr…*
> *You don't have to catheter me,*
> *Doctorrrr…*
> *You don't have to,*
> *Baby, don't put it in…"*

Sharon: Aw, you get to have all the fun.

Greta: If she knows "Roxanne" she's not 14.

Linda: Lol — you get a nurse younger than your heart.

Victoria: At least it wasn't from *Frozen.*
Ruby: Were you wearing that dress again?

Technically, yes. A gown, anyway.

5/23/19
5th heart biopsy completely negative.
So the only thing my heart rejects is the Trump administration.

Kate: When are they going to be done poking your new heart?

Me: Another in 2 weeks, then it goes to once a month they decide that the rejection is stable. After that it's either annually or they just go with a blood test.

5/24/19
2 months ago I couldn't get through half of the "Now is the winter of our discontent" speech without stopping to gasp for air. Today my new-heart-self recited that, "To be or not to be", and Sonnet 18 (twice) all together non-stop. The dog I was walking seemed to wonder what the heck I was doing. #everyone'sacritic

"To be or not to be" was the running theme of my spring, after that discontented cardiac winter I had.

Calling the heart Archie McThump-Thump may have been premature. 'Bob New-heart' may have been the superior choice.

It's of some concern to me that one of the readings on my cardiac rehab monitor is called Final Rest.

Jim: Better than "End of Line."

Marisa: ♫ "It's the final count-down…"

Maria: Yeah. We need a naming contest on this one, I think.

So…I have mild autism (Asperger's) and have an extremely limited tolerance for change. In the past 12 months we sold the house and moved here (1 year tomorrow) and upgraded my heart. And now school is making me move my classroom of 15 years so Health class can have my space. My new space being a newly constructed wonder-room that's not across from the Band Room only helps a tiny bit.

Julie: But it's a NEW ROOM! No drafts! No leaks! No band would be a huge plus for me.

Grace: That sounds like a move up to me. When I was teaching 7th grade Language Arts, I had a room beside the auditorium. The band, chorus, and theater classes would use it. OMG.

Julie: Also new has to have less germs.

True, but probably more formaldehyde and other new-construction poisons. Though if I expire of that, at least I'll leave a presentable body.

Maria: Did you tell them they were really pushing it?

Me: Their $10 million renovation trumps anything mere teachers might want.

Taryn: Awww. I loved that classroom!

Marion: Isn't there some "heart transplant patient returning to work" card you can pull?

Keeping that in reserve for an even-more-irritating event. Always conserve your ammo.

5/25/19
Attending graduation in 2 1/2 hours in my faculty gown and Master's hood. This should make some jaws drop there. All I need is a big-brimmed hat, sunglasses, a bottle of water, and about 3 gallons of SPF 900 sun block.

Rebecca: Don't forget your mask.

Sshhh! You aren't supposed to let them know I'm Batman.

Marisa: Honoring Terry Kroenung, whose heart has graduated from his body and is here today walking.

While the school band plays "Pomp and Circulation."

Beth: Tape a red heart on your gown.

Barbara: Maybe carry a Mylar balloon shaped like a red heart.

*Yeah, the parents sitting behind me who couldn't take photos of their little darling would be **really** forgiving about that.*

Sarah: Should have brought a big parasol!

"Heroic heart transplant survivor slain by enraged camera-wielding mob."

Made it through the graduation speeches, but chose to exercise discretion in the heat and head home once they started handing out the diplomas. Sitting in a black polyester robe in the sun was beginning to become a strain.

Scott: Wise man. I was never a fan of outdoor ceremonies.

Kelly: So were you center of attention when you were there?

*I'm **always** the center of attention...just not usually for the right reason.*

Samantha: I saw you at the beginning of the ceremony but didn't get the chance to say hi.

Maria: You could have stripped naked and walked out in front of everyone, what would they do? You could just yell, "Shut up, suckers! I almost died!"

Me: Me naked would be a war crime prosecuted at the Hague.

Maria: Same defense, of course.

I didn't have that much sunblock with me.

Scott: "Good speaker? He had me in stitches!"

The 24 pills a day are no treat for my stomach. I'm on Protonix and Zantac twice a day to mitigate it. Plus Tums. Plenty of it. I'm eating more chalk than a pre-schooler.

Cynthia: Be careful you don't get stopped up, if you know what I mean and I think you do. Tums is mostly chalk, and can stop you up in a New York minute.

Mark: Try green mint tea.

Curtis: I put my patients with GERD on popcorn, large amount of fiber in popcorn seems to help. And ginger chews help, as well. Calcium is one of the substances that releases acid in the stomach, so Tums buffering is typically very temporary. Mylanta or Maalox is better.

I've gone to swallowing our old kitchen sponges. Waste not…

5/26/19
The Perceived Effort Scale for exertion that I have to go by, having no vagus nerve any more to talk to the heart, is called the Borg Scale. Prepare to be assimilated, heart. Resistance is useless.

New heart went in 7 weeks ago tonight.

5K walk this a.m. 48 minutes. 15:25/mile. Average pulse 125. Max pulse 133.

Hey, you don't buy a Ferrari and then just leave it in the garage.

Looks like I'm officially a regular at the pharmacy. Showed up there today and he pulled my meds and handed them to me without a word being said. 'Free', too, since we hit our annual out-of-pocket maximum around February 13.

Maria: Yeah, like at a small-town restaurant, "Will it be the usual, sir?"

"Hit me again, Sam. You know what I like. Prednisone martini, shaken not stirred."

Julie: You are officially a drugstore cowboy now.

5/28/19
Newest post-transplant adventure: beard-trimming with Prednisone tremors.

Kelly: Go to a barber.

Maria: Yeah, let a professional do this for you.

Professionals…pffft! Look what trained professionals with blades already did to me. Scars every-damned-where.

Me: Too late. All done.

Ali: That was very silly! Hope you didn't do it yourself just for the book.

If I was that crazy, I'd have done my own heart transplant. Nothing by halves.

Cerene: So….do you now look like a kid trying to grow his first facial hair? All patchy and uneven?

Me: Nope. All spiffy. So…ha!

Sharon: I have essential tremors and I spill all over myself (not sure why they call them essential).

Because they're essential to your neurologist getting paid?

So many over-the-counter digestive products on the kitchen counter due to the transplant meds that it looks like we mugged the local district tummy-meds salesman.

"Wanted: Caucasian couple, 60's, for armed robbery of a Mylanta van. Should be considered cramped and dangerous."

Since getting home from the transplant (just over 7 weeks), I've taken roughly 1,125 pills. Doing my part to enable pharmaceutical executives to buy bigger Lear jets.

Maria: I think they should be paying you for all the advertisement!

Can they pay me in tacrolimus pills?

Just tripped over the corner of the couch in the dark and landed head-first on the living room floor. That was exciting. Much outraged cussing involved. Slight, brief ache on right temple. None of the incisions or sternum appear to be re-damaged. On the upside, the Apple watch did vibrate and ask me if I was okay after my fall and should it call 911? That was why we spent the extortionate amount of $ on it in the first place.

Ali: Don't do that! At least the wires on your sternum held. In fact, they'll probably never loosen. It's the rest of you that ya gotta take care of. The Apple watch did "good."

Jill: I'm glad you're okay! An injury is the last thing you need!

Oh, I don't know. The transplant scars are under the clothes. I need a dashing piratical head scar to work up the local ladies.

Kelly: Jesus, Terry! Turn on a light!

Marion: Okay. That is the best reason to get an Apple Watch that I've heard so far.

Eileen: So it's the personal On Star. Does it call 911 if you've been people-jacked? (PS: glad you didn't need it to call)

Me: It detects a fall and reacts. If you're people-jacked, you have to call 911 on it yourself.

Which is why Apple needs to build a TASER into the thing. Or a sedative dart gun.

And notice that I made no joke on 'people-jacked', easy as that would've been.

Maria: Now what did you do that for?

Me: To entertain y'all.

Swings inspirometer, shouts to crowd: "Are you not entertained?!"

Maria: And here I thought it was some sort of a sophisticated experiment to verify the gravitational field consistency on planet Earth.

Me: I do that hourly when I inevitably drop shit.

Suzann: Good to hear you are fine. Does that fancy watch not have a light on it like my phone? If you had been knocked out and unable to respond what does it do? Just curious.

Me: It would have called 911 and given them my address and a map to the house.

And then it would've laughed at me for being a clumsy doofus…in a Mickey Mouse voice. "Gee, you're a waste of air, pal."

Sarah: My iPhone always has our house number wrong when it tries to auto-fill. I wonder if I dialed 911, if it would take help to my neighbors.

"Hello, we'd like to share the good news of 'The Watchtower' with you. And might you need a cardiac catheterization while we're here?"

Tim: According to the Mueller report there's NO CONCUSSION!

Me: But there was clearly obstruction, thus the fall.

Bruce: Are you sure it wasn't just telling you it was time to get in your next 300 steps?

"Hey, get off of your lazy ass and jog around the block, sport!"

Read an article about cardiac sarcoidosis. So rare that they have little data or knowledge of the heart form. Maybe 10,000 cases a year out of 320 million people in the U.S. Yeah, I'm special. This is also what happened to me: "Dr. Birnie treated the arrhythmia with a pacemaker and thought nothing more of it — until the same patient returned two years later suffering from heart failure. Upon further investigation, it turned out that she had cardiac sarcoidosis."

Me: "Sarcoidosis is a rare disease, affecting anywhere from five to 64 people in every 100,000; symptoms due to cardiac involvement are present in perhaps 5% of all cases. Unfortunately, right now, there is no way to predict who will have a relatively benign disease and whose disease will progress."

As my wife would say, sighing and rolling her eyes, "Yeah, you're a rarity, all right."

5/29/19
New running shirt, carefully designed to inflict maximum humiliation on the 'norms.' (photo 72)

Suzann: You are so bad.

AE: Oh, you devil you! Not running in any race with you! You'd beat my arse.

Julie: I like your style, and you'd be ahead of me with the old heart!

Maria: I think that font needs to be a bit bigger.

Me: That's as big as I could make it and get all the words in.

Maria: Yeah, but how will they be able to read it as you fade away in the distance?

My vortex will suck them behind me like dry leaves behind the Road Runner. Beep-beep!

5/30/19
Today's 'Delusions of Grandeur' tour:

Tried to run .25 mile as an experiment, after .75 mile warmup. Holy hell. After .05 had to stop, bend over, and suck air for 5 breaths before continuing. Did that 4 more times to get the distance. Pulse up to 135 (the highest I've ever got it up to is 141). Legs and arms felt like gravity had increased several times. Any conditioning I had before is utterly gone and I'm starting totally from scratch.

I found out later that, thanks to the denervation, a lot of conditioning will likely never return.

Carrie: At least you get to start!

Me: Don't tell my doctors. I'm breaking rules.

Hmm…I say that a lot.

Julie: We will keep your secret. /zips lips and throws away the key/

Sarah: I think your body is telling you're only young at heart.

I beg to differ. Janet says I'm completely infantile, so there.

Jacqueline: I think if you're even trying to run, you're winning.

Kelly: I'm gonna tell mom!!

Maria: Don't tell mom. Tell his surgeon.

Kelly: Mom has more clout!

Maria: Okay. Both. Let's have a redundancy — like in engineering.

Maria: You do remember you had a heart transplant surgery like 15 minutes ago, right?

Tim: I ran for the first time today. I ran a mile. I'm definitely out of shape, but this heart is strong.

5/31/19
It's June tomorrow. So this is the last day that I can casually mention, "Oh, yeah. I had a heart transplant just last month."

6/1/19
I'm entered in this for July 21. I'm not messing around with the new heart. Archie needs to get with the program. (photo 73)

With the nagging leg injuries keeping me from training, I ended up having to walk a lot of it. Oh, well…

Mirror, mirror, on the wall, who has the biggest heart of them all? (photo 74)

"The heart of the whale is larger than the pipe of the waterworks at London Bridge. The water in that pipe is not so thick or fast as the blood pumping from the heart of the whale." – 'Moby Dick'

"At an average of 2.4 meters, Blue Whales have the largest penis in the animal kingdom, and their single ejaculation contains 20 liters of sperm." – the Interwebs (that's a hell of an ejection fraction)

I leave it to you, discerning reader, as to which of these is the more impressive.

Sarah: You have very verbose friends.

Maria: Aren't you glad we did all that writing for you?

First rule I learned in the infantry: always get somebody else to expend their ammo on your enemy first.

Marie Kondo said to get rid of anything that didn't give me joy. So I threw my heart away and got a younger one. You know, like Trump does with his wives.

And his Cabinet Secretaries, apparently.

6/2/19
Good news: I can run 1/10 of a mile at an ordinary jogging pace before I have to stop and breathe. That's 3 times as far as last time I tried. Bad news: That's the same distance I could run with advanced heart failure.

Me: #babysteps

Julia: Don't rush things.

Like I have a choice.

Rebecca: How do you know the previous owner exercised? That heart could be begging for mercy.

AE: Maybe it's yer legs, not yer pumper.

Ana: What's the rush? Life is not a marathon, it's a journey.

Scott: It's because he prepared for a marathon that he now has some laps left to go.

Richard: BUT then you were on the way down and NOW you're on the way back UP!!

Today's marital bonding experience: driving around town loading up on disinfectant wipes, Lysol spray, Zantac, and Mylanta to deal with my immunosuppression issues. #loveneverdies

Maria: Ahhh, romance is in the air!

As is the smell of medicinal alcohol.

I'm happy to report that I have a mild right calf strain...from running! #Icallthatprogress

AE: Well done. Crutches now????

Kelly: Karma! Running without doctors' okay!

6/3/19
Before-and-after chest x-ray of a pacemaker patient who received a heart transplant, showing the permanent wires holding the sternum together. 6 days after transplant. (photo 75)

Rebecca: You got some long lungs, better warn the techs before the picture.

Me: They often have to take 3 descending shots and combine them.

Rebecca: I have done that too many times. Warning them helps.

Cerene: We can see INSIDE you. That is really neat to see!

Me: That's different. Usually people say they can see THROUGH me.

6/4/19
I've solved my problem with immunosuppressive infection. (photo 76)

I guess I shouldn't complain about my many hospital issues.

(headline) "Flash fire ignites in man's chest during emergency heart surgery." (link # 9)

It's literal heartburn!

Did they put it out with a Zantac fire extinguisher?

6/5/19
It's a bit ironic that my leg still hurts too much to go to the hospital gym for rehab.

Just had a 4-sneeze fit and it didn't hurt. #fearmysternum

6/6/19
At the medical center for another cardiac biopsy. If all is negative, they should be only doing them once a month from now on. Pity. I so look forward to these cozy familial jugular vein stabbings.

It seems a bit cruel that the door to the hospital billing office is in the waiting room of the blood draw center.

Sessha: It is like that at our hospital, too. I wonder if someone in hospital design has a wicked sense of humor.

Ana: And that's not even 1/10th of the entire billing staff; some of the coders, and those that collect and verify insurance and responsible party info billing, are in an unmarked building off of Lowry.

One imagines them getting to work via a mile-long hallway of blast doors and then dropping down a phone booth elevator.

And if you can't be bothered to recognize the opening credits scene of 'Get Smart!', then I'm sorry, we can't be friends. #standards

I was doing this a year ago, and here I am now using somebody else's heart. (photo 77)

Jacqueline: Crazy to think your ticker was already very ill and you didn't know. So glad you're still here to tell the tale!

Bad news, world: I'm still here because I'm the new herald of Galactus.

Galactus: Planet-eating entity in Marvel comics. The amount of Mylanta he consumes boggles the mind.

My BNP test of cardiac stress is now in the green range. 100 or below is normal. In mid-March it was 900. That indicates advanced heart failure. Now I'm all healed-ish and the new heart is no longer complaining about its new condo.

It is complaining about the asshat landlord, though.

So...it's 10 am and I'm lying on a gurney waiting for my 9:30 am biopsy.

Kelly: It's been 2 weeks already?

Me: Yep.

Paul: Only twenty-three and a half hours to go!

Barbara: It's hurry up and wait at every hospital.

Me: Hilariously, they told me as they were removing the catheter from my neck that they were trying to streamline the waiting system and how was my hospital experience today?

Today's biopsy playlist: I requested "My Heart Will Go On", just to be a smartass, and the nurse refused to play it (a lady of taste and refinement, Kat is). So we went with show tunes. As the procedure started, needles in the neck, it was "Can You Feel the Love Tonight?" from *The Lion King*. As it ended, they played "Somewhere Over the Rainbow" and "Defying Gravity" back-to-back. So I had talking lions, munchkins, and witches.

Jim: At least you didn't get "My Friends" from *Sweeney Todd*.

"A Little Priest" would've been worse.

Paul: "Take Another Little Piece of My Heart?" "Bits and Pieces?" "Needles and Pins?" "I Lost My Heart to a Starship Trooper?" "Keep the Customer Satisfied"?

♫ *"The first cut is the deepest..."*

My tacrolimus trough reading today is 13.7. Top that!

Courtney: I would try to top that if I knew what the heck you were saying.

Me: The anti-rejection med blood test is perfect.

Got a little too smug a little too soon on that one.

Guess who's medically cleared for running and biking? This guy, that's who.

Scott: Did they clear you, or just come to the inevitable realization that they couldn't stop you?

Me: Back off. I have it in writing.

Theresa: I do agree, though, you seem an unstoppable force. Thanks be to younger hearts and good surgeons.

Sharon: I think he's lying...

Grace: Woot! Back to the bike!

Ana: You missed the BolderBoulder this year!

I'm betting they didn't miss me, though.

So when I asked if I could get on the bike, the studly *Grey's Anatomy*-level cardiologist shoved on my chest like he was doing last-ditch CPR and said, "You're fine."

Ali: What happens if a recent heart surgery patient did need CPR? Presumably not the best idea with a recently sawn sternum? Is that why they leave pacing wires in?

Me: The pacing wires only stay in about 3 days.

They're already starting to taper-down my Prednisone.

Sorry, mighty Prednisone Corporation, you'll have to suck your massive profits somewhere else.

Actually, it's an old generic drug that costs next to nothing compared to the other immunosuppressants. So at least I'm not getting economically gouged while getting poisoned by it.

The biopsy doctor wore a vest over his scrubs with cartoon T-rexes on it. Said it was his spirit animal. I told him that didn't inspire confidence in his ability to perform a fine vascular/cardiac procedure on me.

Ana: And you were not afraid he was going to spit in your port before poking you?

I just assumed every doctor already did that.

Cerene: I dunno...big head, tiny hands...seems legit.

♫ **"Tacrolimus, my old friend...I had to swallow you again...This is the sound...of transplant..."**

Me: That med sounds like a Roman general.

Lisa: Caius Martius Tacrolimus!

Me: "Besides suppressing the immune response that could lead to acute cellular rejection, organ failure, and death, what have the Romans ever done for us?"

From Monty Python's 'Life of Brian.' I tried to think of a reason to use the 'Biggus Dickus' bit, but it was a, um, stretch. I would've had to go to great lengths to fit it in.

6/7/19
Potential transplant book title: *Lost Vagus: Don't gamble with your cardiac health.*

Heart transplant was 2 months ago today. I'm about to go out on the bike for the first time since forever.

Rebecca: Watch for potholes, you don't need that.

That means something else in Colorado now.

10 miles on the bike. Woo-hoo! Cruising speed about the same as before the transplant, but the legs are dead, dead, dead. And the neck is so weak now it's hard to keep my head up. Got up a 6% hill okay.

Another perfect biopsy result, zero rejection. Off to pick up the new Prednisone prescription to start tapering that from 20 mg to 16 mg. 20% less of it a day can only be a good thing.

6/8/19
At 1 a.m. the iPad chimed nonstop, freaking out the basset hound. It was 47 e-mailed medical bills.

Julie: Dogs always sense danger.

Liana: Is your calculator smoking?

Andrea: It would be nice if medical organizations gave you opportunity to fully recover first before they started the barrage.

Me: Oh, they've been arriving forever. Technically, they aren't bills, because we reached our out-of-pocket maximum a long time ago. We don't have to pay them, but the insurance company does.

Andrew: This is one thing that never happens here. And I'm glad and appreciate what we have. It scares me that 45 and his pals want to get their grubby mitts on this country's proudest institution. I have to hope against hope that it never happens.

Hopefully he'll be **in** *an institution first.*

6/9/19
I just sanitized a telephone. Help me, I'm on the B Ark.

Yeah, yeah, yeah, more 'Hitchhiker's Guide to the Galaxy' stuff.

Garalt: Get that hot tub practice in now.

Me: You're never lonely when you have a rubber duck.

Eric: The only thing keeping humanity alive, it turns out.

An enormous mutant star goat!

Working back up to running again after twinging the calf a week ago. 5K walk at 15:39/mile. No problem with leg or new heart.

Maria: When are you coming to Zumba?!

When I've finished my commitment to training Olympic rock climbers. Priorities…

6/10/19
Still transcribing transplant FB posts/comments into the book document.

Garalt: Does this book have an appendix, at least?

Me: No, it went bad and the surgeons removed it.

About to bail on cardiac rehab. I don't need babysitters. It's not like they actually supervise me. All they do is check my blood pressure and turn me loose. I can run and bike on my own. I have an elliptical machine in my house, along with a BP cuff, O2 sensor, thermometer, and pulse monitor. And everybody needs to get off my ass about this. I was a fully trained Army physical fitness trainer, designing plans like this every day. I know when my time is being wasted. My personal workouts are much harder and better for me. 10 minutes on a treadmill does nothing.

Sure enough, the cardiologists all agreed that it was wasting my time and canceled it.

Tapering down the Prednisone from 20 mg to 18. So now I'm at about 30 pills a day.

AE: You druggie, you! Tapering is good!

Julie: Hey, less meds is less! Will you eventually be totally off the Prednisone?

Me: That was the original plan, but now that sarcoidosis is confirmed, they'll have to leave it at 5 mg to prevent it from coming back.

Robin: Assume you have tried cannabis oil for your ailments?

Me: Can't. Interferes with the rejection meds. Transplant Team said no.

Alaena: They probably check. It's pretty hard core and specific instructions. Natural is usually better, but when you have spare parts it's probably not advisable to go off protocol. They have to follow their patients for life, and want to know all the details as each person is their own case study.

My weight in gold: $3,336,000. Or not even 2 heart transplants.

Richard: Goodness! Figuring $1300 an ounce, I'd cost $4,846,400!

One instance where dining at the all-you-can-eat buffet literally pays off.

6/11/19
Day I on the reduced Prednisone dose. We'll see if the side effects fall noticeably, too. In 2 weeks it goes down again.

Spoiler: they did not.

12 miles on the road bike. Faster than Friday, legs not as dead, despite the late rehab session yesterday. About 4:30/mile for the first

10, which is only :30/mile slower than before the transplant. Out again Thursday, to share my spandexed backside with the world.

Clearly, I post too much transplant stuff on here. Facebook just gave me an ad for stethoscopes.

Sharon: You make my day!

Pete: Please don't stop. It would be disheartening.

I see what you did there.

Sean: I'll have you know *I* just got a stethoscope ad because I laughed at your post.

6/12/19
5K power walk in 44:44. 14:24/mile. Better than 4 mph. That's all I could ever do before, so I'm declaring myself 'cured' as far as walking goes.

At least for the cardiovascular system. The leg muscles blow out if you just give them a cruel glare.

Tried jogging again, after letting the dodgy calf heal. Didn't hurt this time. Still don't have any endurance yet (only been 9 1/2 weeks since the transplant). Can just only manage 1/10 of a mile, then have to take 10 deep breaths and go again for another 1/10. Did 5 of those at a 9:36/mile pace. 6 weeks till the organ donors 5K race/fun run I signed up for. Hopefully the conditioning starts to come back at a faster rate so I don't have to do it on a gurney.

Julie: You're already better than me.

Alaena: You could just walk it and finish the darn thing faster than probably the bottom 1/3 of the participants, I'm guessing.

Maria: I can only manage 1/10 of a mile — period. And I haven't had a heart transplant.

Me: You should get one. All the cool kids are doing it.

Maria: Sure, I'll just pop over to the local outlets.

'Organs R Us.'
'Wal-Heart.'
'Chestco'

Spotted what I thought was a used condom on our coffee table. This would be problematic and highly unlikely for innumerable reasons. As I'm A) wondering who broke into our house to shag on our table and B) looking for 27 Lysol wipes and a tanker truck of Purell, it finally dawned on me what it really was. A cheese stick wrapper.

Julie: You have a man brain.

Maria: Do you need an eye transplant, too?

Me: I DO have cataracts.

Fiona: It amuses me highly to think that the thought that Janet may have another man in never crossed your mind! Mind you, if the size of a cheese straw wrapper...not worth the bother!

Julie: That's what my husband said. Lololol

Maria: Is that a cheese straw in your pocket, or are you happy to see me?

Me: Janet is overwhelmed by me. No energy for a bit on the side. Just sayin'.

Transplant Team says I only have to do two sessions a week for two more weeks and I'm done, since I'm already doing workouts way beyond theirs. So ha!, doubters.

Stephany: Now, now, no need to get all superior, just because you survived a deadly heart and have turned into Superman.

"Faster than a speeding wheelchair…more powerful than an MRI scan…able to leap tall Outpatient Pavilions in a single bound…"

Pulse on the brief run this a.m. got up to 164. Theoretically that's higher than the old heart could go before it started to die. #yougoArchie

6/13/19
15 miles on the bike today. Slow, but got it done. Building the miles a little at a time. Right leg a bit shinplinty from yesterday's fast 5K walk and brief run, but the cycling motion didn't really bother it. Muscles still resistant, not in the old shape yet, but still managed a 22-mph acceleration to beat a yellow light.

Let me tell you how much harder it is to run a yellow light on a bike than in a car…

Maria: You know, if you end up at the same hospital because you'd fallen off your bike and broken something, your entire transplant will come down and beat you — as well they should.

Me: They said I could ride the bike.

Julie: They had no idea you meant 15 miles. I'd bet green money on that one.

Garalt: Only the heart is less than your age…remember that. Don't break out the slippers yet, but you're one of the more driven people I know, and chilled out dudes tend to live longer, just sayin'.

Dead dudes are literally more chilled.

6/14/19
♬ **"I left my heart…in Denver's OR…"**

Giselle: Now write the rest of the lyrics.

Me: ♫ "More than three times, it tried to kill me.
                    Full of sarcoid, it left me with scars
                    Nearly from chin to knee."

Dave: How they fixed your "off-beat" humor?

Nanci: Theme song: "I Got Rhythm."

Me: "The Beat Goes On."

Nanci: With my irregular heartbeat, mine is "All That Jazz."

Remember, always give 100%.
Unless you're doing a live liver donation. Then you might want to
settle for 50%.

6/15/19
My daily hors d'oeuvres. 36 hits a day. Most of it is to counteract the
side effects of the top row.

Top row, **L to R, morning: Mycophenelate mofetil, for rejection (at**
night, too). Tacrolimus, for rejection (at night, too). 15 mg
Prednisone, for rejection. 3 mg Prednisone (combined for 18 mg,
tapering from 20 mg toward 16 mg and beyond this).

Middle row, **L to R: Calcium/Vitamin D, for osteoporosis prevention**
from the meds (at night, too). Sulfamethoxazole-trimethoprim, for
pneumocystis jiroveci pneumonia prevention (3 times a week,
M/W/F). Low-dose aspirin, blood thinner for heart health.
Amlodipine, to prevent high blood pressure. Forgot to lay out the
Bupropion, for depression.

Bottom row, **L to R, night only: Valgoncivlovir, to prevent**
cytomegalovirus. Prevastatin, to prevent hyperlipidemia.

Levothyroxine, for my pre-existing hyperthyroidism. Bottle at right: Nystatin, to prevent thrush infection (4 times a day).

<u>Also</u>: 2 Ranitidine, 2 multivitamins, 2 fish oil, 2 fiber gummies. (photo 78)

150 pages & 40,000 words on the transplant book so far. That's still not with all of the comments on my FB posts added in. Only up to May 1 on those. Then the actual writing begins, with Janet and I making observations/explanations on what happened.

6/16/19
Another heart transplant observation:
If your condition fascinates every doctor who hears about it, that is NOT necessarily a good thing.

The worst is having a disease named after you. That never ends well.

Hopefully everyone is having a splendid Father's Day. That said...There's a donor father somewhere in New Mexico who's having probably the worst one of his life. #thanksdadwhoeveryouare

Julie: I believe that the fact that he saved someone else — maybe lots of others — will help him.

Helen: I wondered when you would mention him. Don't get me wrong, I am 100% happy for you but all along I have been struggling with...a 19-year-old...

Cindi: Being the former wife of a donor, it was the gift of life to someone in need that helped us feel somewhat comforted after James' accident. He was 29, but still so young. Happy that he lives on still in those he helped.

6/17/19
Today's Amazon suggestions: a book on atrial fibrillation, a hydroponics kit, and stuff for turning my fireplace flame into pretty

colors. Apparently, because of the Colorado address and the cardiac issues, they think I need to take my mind off of my failing heart by smoking my own home-grown weed while staring into a Technicolor fire. #theyaren'tfarwrong

AE: Well...do you??? Is Amazon right?

Me: Can't do the demon weed, even if I wanted to. Interferes with the rejection meds.

Alaena: The technicolor fire is kinda cool, but not for a gas fireplace or even indoors for that matter. Lots of health warning on the package.

Tina: I had a strong afib episode this morning. Don't need a book, sadly, know all about it!

6/19/19
Jumped out of bed this morning and got so light-headed I had to grab the bathroom counter to keep from falling over. Clearly the 19-year-old heart hates getting up early, like all teenagers.

Ana: Well, yeah, it's summer break!

AE: Solution: sleep till noon.

Maybe I need to take up gaming and saying, "Dude!" a lot.

Transplant book formatting is underway.

Jim: "It was a dark and stormy night. Suddenly, a heart attack rang out!" *"Sing, O Muse, of the wrath of the patient."*

6/20/19
Because I haven't fully plumbed the depths of the medical abyss, I now have an appointment to get knocked out and have a camera shoved down my mouth and nearly out the other end. That must be why they call it an endoscope.

Christine: Hope had one done from the top, and one done from the bottom to assess the damage done by her IBS. She asked the doctor, with great trepidation, if they did the endoscopy before the colonoscopy. He laughed, said everyone asks that, and assured her they used two different scopes for the two different procedures.

Mark: It's an easy one. Had it a few years back and I was sitting up having a cuppa tea and a sandwich ten minutes after waking up.

Kat: I sympathize. I have a similar appointment on 31 July. Mine differs slightly in that they're also going in through my ileostomy too. At the same time. Thus the general anesthetic. We shall have to support one another with jokes in deplorable taste!

Deplorable taste? "Child, you cut me to the quick!" (Frank Morgan in 'The Wizard of Oz.')

Rebecca: It's the prep that is miserable. I am coming up on 10 years so I am due. Had no idea how fast Gatorade went through the body.

About as fast as a real gator would.

Bren: In one endo and out the othero!

Pop the champagne! Amazon just sent me a royalty notice for...wait for it...$4.12. Yee-haw!

Julie: It was not a bill. Good enough!

Fiona: If you added a couple of dollars, you could at least get a bottle of Prosecco!

Or a bottle of Mylanta.

Julia: My royalties this month will be the highest I've ever gotten from Amazon — $36 in one month. WOW!

Serge: Party! Party! Party!

Mandy: More than I have ever got from them!!

Maria: Don't spend it all in one place.

Tina: Dinner's on you, right?

I'm so clumsy, dinner's always 'on' me.

6/22/19
Current total for all of this transplant stuff: $1,000,407.28. We paid $4,000 and owe no more.

That total looked positively meagre later.

Me: Quality school district health insurance.

Joshwa: I may need to switch plans.

Joe: And you can thank the ACA for not having a $1,000,000 lifetime cap!

Cindy: I'm glad for you. Also terrified that my plan isn't so good.

I'm here to tell you, few things are more disturbing than hearing MS Word robotically read your phrase "they cut my heart out and threw it in a trash can" like Stephen Hawking.

Dave: With that faint note of robotic glee...

I'd rather it sound like Marvin the Paranoid Android: "I think you ought to know that I'm feeling very depressed..." (there's a Douglas Adams quote for every occasion)

"Your plastic pal who's fun to be with!"

6/23/19
Heart transplant was 11 weeks ago tonight. 77 days. I suppose those lucky 7's are appropriate.

6/24/19
Sitting in a hospital as a mere visitor. Not having anything injected, sliced, or removed. Don't know how to behave.

Me: Janet would say that I've NEVER known how to behave. #fairenough

Me: She's getting a routine blood draw.

Cynthia: It's like going to someone else's party, isn't it?

♬ *"It's my party and I'll bleed if I wanna…"*

Me: I'll be back at my transplant center tomorrow, though, getting a baseline skin cancer screening, since the meds increase the risk 10X.

As of today, I'm on 20% less Prednisone than I started with.

(checks pockets) I know I had it here someplace…

Me: It's the little things.

Me: Hands still shaking. Probably shouldn't be disarming any bombs quite yet.

Tim: I'm down to 5mg per day as of last week. Not a whole lotta shaking going on anymore.

Me: That will be my end point, because of the sarcoidosis.
Tim: I'm fortunate enough that I'll likely be off completely at some point.

6/25/19
Off to my transplant hospital again, to the Cancer Pavilion.
Just getting a baseline skin cancer exam, since my risk is 10X higher when immunosuppressed. 2-hour round trip for a 20-minute visit. #thefunneverends

Adam: Isn't there an app for that?

Me: 11 different specialists don't get paid if you do that.

Just had liquid nitrogen sprayed on the top of my bald head. That was new and different. Zapping some possibly pre-cancerous spots, in an abundance of caution. Otherwise, I'm good for a year.

Should've sung, "♫ The cold never bothered me anyway..."

Nancy: It's an interesting feeling. I kept reminding myself it wasn't *hot,* it was very *cold*.

Maria: When I was in fifth grade and we were studying thermodynamics in our physics class, our instructor dropped a rubber ball into a container with liquid nitrogen, then picked it out with tongs, dropped it, and let it shatter. It was to demonstrate that we should not stick our fingers or any other body parts into liquid nitrogen. Very educational.

Ah, that zany Soviet school system...

Ana: Does it turn your brain into ice cream?

Me: Too late.

Eileen: Yeah, the Irish girl here is an old acquaintance of the canister. It's particularly fun on your cheek (the one under your eyes.)

Sharon: Adds new meaning to "brain freeze!"

Serge: You're now Mr. Freeze? Holy villain, Batman!

I'd rather be the Penguin. I already have the top hat, umbrella, spats, tux, and monocle for that. (Gawd, I need a life)

Ah, public restrooms. Or as we immunosuppressed think of them, 'suicide caverns.' #notenoughpurellintheworld

6/26/19
Just did 20 miles on the bike, now that the @#$! rain and wind have finally stopped and my leg doesn't hurt. No cardiac or other problems. Archie McThump-Thump's just fine with it.

At least, he seems to be. Pretty sure his way of complaining would be a real attention-getter.

My new bike jersey arrived today. SPF 35. It perfectly describes my cycling. The back of the collar says "I used to be faster." And the latest, and likely last, snarky transplant shirt came, too. (photos 79, 80)

Dai: Can't you get one that says, "Old Fart, New Heart"?

6/27/19
Why is my heart so slow to respond after the transplant? I haven't the vagus idea.

Me: I'll see myself out...

Cynthia: I'll hold the door.

Cerene: Thank for having the heart to tell us. We're all pumped now.

Serge: You're fired!

Julie: Where is the eye-roll button?

Dave: There's your off-"beat" humor again!

Veronica: So good I nearly shit my pants. (Because the vagus nerve controls the viscera, too.)

That probably explains my decidedly irregular intestinal episodes now.

Lisa: It takes a lot of nerve to make a pun like that.

6/28/19
Total medical bills since January 1: $1,840,513.29 That's enough to stop the new heart in its tracks.

Julie: I thought it would be a lot more! Ours were at 7 figures when my husband almost cut his leg off with a chainsaw.

Me: First off: ouch. Second, it's still counting. It's around $20,000 every time I get a biopsy.

Maria: Well... We already established you didn't do anything halfway.

Well, halfway would be 'old heart removed and...stop.'

Theresa: Keep going. Almost to the 6 million mark.

Pretty sure the rates have gone up since the 1970's.

AE: What's the twenty-nine cents all about? At this point, they should just round.

The amounts are always weird like that. I'm surprised they don't bill in shekels or pieces of eight.

Sharon: And the new heart changes from ba-da-bump...to ka-ching...

6/30/19
Nothing wrong with me that about $4000 worth of bike and equipment can't cure.

Me: With that new old fart jersey, drivers certainly don't have the excuse that they couldn't see me coming.

I've had people stop me so they could take pictures of the jersey.

Another 20 miles on the bike without incident. Might've gone a little farther, but it was 95 degrees at that point and discretion conquered valor.

I'm going back through all of the transplant FB posts and comments as I prepare this crazy book. So far, I've found 3 people who honestly/seriously/no joke <u>offered to donate half their livers or a kidney to me</u> if that had been necessary. One was a college theatre department friend, another a former student. One was somebody I'd never actually been in the same room with and only know through FB.

Me: Just to be clear, this is volunteering for major, dangerous surgery that takes months to recover from.

Joshwa: I would have done it, too, though my liver is no good to anyone, after what I've put it through.

*Remember: if it doesn't kill you, it will make you stronger…but it **will** still piss you off.*

Greta: That's an extraordinary offer, Terry. Wow.

S.F.: Should have taken them up on it. All of them. 2 and 1/2 livers!

Scott: Sounds like a sitcom!

That would actually be a more accurate title for '2 ½ Men.'

Cue the "Live Organ Transplants" scene again.

To access the photos/videos/links:
www.terrykroenungink.com/246-2/

7) Snarkoidosis

August 1-September 8, 2019

And here we get toward the end of our little snarkfest. I arbitrarily chose to end it when I resumed teaching and attended a block party on our street, as that seemed like a significant, upbeat victory. The students didn't seem nearly as thrilled for the new school year as I was. Maybe it was just the end of their carefree summer, but it could've also have been all of the mandatory hand and desk sanitizing I insisted on. With so much hand rubbing, they probably felt like Lady Macbeth talking to her dog: "Out, damned spot!"

This section covers all of July, starting with my 12th-week marking of the transplant, and goes to mid-August and teaching high school again at the 4-month mark. July started off with my cycling distance increasing to 50 kilometers (30 miles) as a high, and a white blood cell count in the sub-basement as a low. That last one, coupled with long-term intestinal outrages that would be crimes against humanity if weaponized, had the Transplant Team test me for all manner of potentially fatal infections. At least those, and the biopsies, remained positively negative.

*The running remained a sore spot, literally. I went from shin splints and calf strains in June to a groin strain in July (yeah, yeah, get the sniggering out of your system), so not much training happened except on the bike. When I did jog, it was like climbing a mountain of wet sand with a Buick on my back. Slow, slow, slow. And I had to stop every 1/10 mile to breathe. But it began to gradually improve. When I could go ¼ mile without stopping, I felt like Rocky on top of the Philly steps (I **looked** like a particularly old and unwell zombie that had originally perished from chain-smoking). But I did manage to stagger through the Donor Dash 5K in Denver in late July, running 2 of the 3 miles, 250 steps at a time. At times it felt like I'd end up an organ donor before reaching the finish line.*

7/1/19
12 weeks ago today this is what I was doing. (photo 81)

Now I'm doing this. #qualitydoctoring (photo 82)

Sessha: I assume this is NOT a picture from today?

Me: Yeah, I had all of that equipment moved into my house out of sheer nostalgia.

Veronica: Quality patienting.

Ana: Now you have a bed with two wheels and it won't let you fall asleep.

Didn't sleep in the hospital with 4-on-the-floor, either, though admittedly the risk of collision with a pickup truck was a tad lower.

Just got back from the 24-hour hospital pharmacy with a grocery bag full of meds, as you do.

A guy there waiting for his meds asked me, in all seriousness, if they put a pig heart in me. It was all I could do to not stutter like Porky the Pig, "Are you insa—insa—insa—uh, crazy?"

Ana: Did you have "any questions for the pharmacist"?

That pops up on the screen every time you're there, when you're signing for your controlled substances.

And why Prednisone is a controlled substance when it causes uncontrolled tremors is another of life's little mysteries.

Me: I almost started off with "Why were we born, only to suffer and die?" and then progress to the phenomenology of mind and Cartesian dualism, but the pharmacist didn't look to be in a forgiving mood.

Mark: Well, that's dinner sorted.

(meme) "Dr. Frankenstein entered a bodybuilding competition and discovered that he had seriously misunderstood the objective."

But the Monster did win Mr. Universe. He was jacked.

7/2/19
25 miles on the bike and all is right with the world (and the heart, lungs, and legs). The head may be up for debate. Haven't been able to do that many miles since October 28 last year.

Eat my dust, terminal heart failure!

7/3/19
Maybe YOU observe Independence Day with fireworks and cookouts, but I settle for nothing less than a cardiac biopsy through my jugular vein. You can have your beer. I'm getting Lidocaine today.

Veronica: You're too cool for me.

Me: It's a curse.

Jim: I got some Lido this past Monday, dude. That's some good shit.

Me: I'm just getting a dab in the neck to dull the catheter site.

Jim: Yeah, it was a dab in the wrist for the IV insert.

Ana: It's amazing! I got some a few months ago. My butt never felt happier. Too bad it doesn't last longer.

"My butt never felt happier." This sounds like a story that would probably boost this book's sales. Please, continue.

Me: Fentanyl, however, is just plain terrifying in its wonderfulness.

It's Franz Kafka's birthday and I'm sitting in an enormous and impersonal institution waiting to have my body invaded with sharp medical instruments.

Julie: Maybe a big cockroach will sit next to you in the waiting room.

Me: That would at least enliven the wait.

You know, diarrhea while waiting for your cardiac biopsy actually isn't the carnival fun ride everybody says it is. #yetanotherTMIevent

Me: Janet's dealing with it, too, so it's not a transplant issue.

Mark: Musta been that dinner. Complain to the pharmacist about storing their pills at the wrong temperature.

Maria: No? Who knew?

And, as usual, the biopsy's 30 minutes late and counting.

If a biopsy ever happens on time, they may have to defibrillate me again.

In the good news/bad news arena:

Good: 0% rejection again on the heart.

Bad: Due to the Montezuma's Revenge-type issue, which has a very slight chance of being CMV (cytomegalovirus, very nasty, possibly fatal, if you have no immune system), I get to spend my 4th of July producing & preparing a poop sample & taking it down to the local hospital.

Update: All negative for CMV.

The irony is that the fantasy novels I write all have at least one scene with animated poop attacking our intrepid young heroine. Thank the gods that life didn't imitate art in my bathroom.

Mark: How many times do they do rejection tests before they decide your body will keep the new heart? It seems to me it's already accepted it, I would think.

Me: At least 6 months. If it stays at zero, they may move to a blood test instead of punching holes in me.

The Transplant Team says the price of Archie beating is eternal vigilance. You can be fine for years and then boom! rejection creeps in.

Cerene: Well, crap. That's a shitty holiday.

Shouldn't it be "Well, crap: that's a shitty holiday"? That sentence really needs a, um, colon.

Unless I need surgery there, then it'd require a semi-colon.

Everything was mostly fine on this month's biopsy/clinic, but...

My white blood cell count is now half of what it was a month ago (from 4.0 to 1.9), and it was marginal then. It's now considered 'problematic' (neutropenic). Because that basically means they've overcooked the rejection meds and now my immune system has gone the way of the dodo and the moderate Republican. I'm VERY prone to infection right now.

So I just had to rearrange the pills in my weekly bin thingie, because the mycophenolate is going to half what it is now, the tacrolimus is going up a fraction, and the Prednisone is coming down again.

Me: The cardiologist (with his charming German accent) making the decisions said not to worry, "You aren't the first."

Sarah: Less Prednisone. That's good. I wonder if it is your wonder athlete status...in that most people that have organ transplants aren't as active as you. Which effects the metabolism of the drugs...my 2 pennies.

Me: I blame Trump.

To be honest, I blame Trump for the Great Depression, the Black Death, and the Punic Wars.

Johnnie: You're Superman. I'm not worried.

Me: Yeah, but there's this Kryptonite thing...

Johnnie: Stay away from that stuff!

I tried, but I'm pretty certain that it was what they used for my 3 nuclear amyloidosis tests.

Today's biopsy song du jour: "Tiny Dancer" by Elton John. So I got to hear "Lay me down in sheets of linen" while doing basically that. My heart got to be the guinea pig/classroom for a newbie who was being coached by the head doctor. Once he scraped the inside of the heart so hard, it felt like a finger jabbed the inside of my chest. I almost went airborne off the table. But the neck site doesn't hurt like the last couple, so at least he's smooth on that front.

The nurses were overseeing this while discussing 'Toy Story 4.'

*Apropos of nothing: Is it inappropriate here to point out that the mom in those movies bought her kid toys named Buzz and Woody? What's up with **that**, Mom? Is hubby not holding up his end?*

Yes, I was walking around the Cardiac Unit in my 'Transplant scars are sexy, wanna see?' T-shirt today. It was a hit. I may have sold a bunch of them indirectly, the staff were so amused. Amazon's getting even richer now.

Well, they are sexy...if your tastes run toward romantic encounters in a morgue.

7/4/19
A week from today Janet gets a colonoscopy, general anesthesia, in the morning. In the afternoon, at the same hospital, I get an endoscopy, general anesthesia, thus completing our whirlwind tour

of the alimentary canal. **Our 17th anniversary is the next day. Who says we don't know how to keep the spark alive?**

Me: Just hoping that they don't use her instrument on me, too.

Cindi: After 17 years you probably share a biome.

Me: 21, counting the 4 years of glorious pre-marital shacking up.

Janet: I think we've absorbed a good portion of basset hound DNA, also.

It's a miracle we haven't contracted brown lung disease from all of the shedding.

(Nasty lung issue seen in textile workers, from inhaling cotton dust)

Andrew: I get my colonoscopy with a little pain killer. It's slightly uncomfortable but not that bad. This time (my third) I wasn't even aware after the first few seconds of anything at all. I've had the same doctor each time. I think she's getting better at it. Endoscopy, however, is a different matter. I had one once and wish I'd been asleep through it. Best wishes.

Me: They didn't give us any other option.

Sharon: Who's the designated driver?

Me: Mr. McGoo.

Yeah, there's a reference nobody under 55 will get.

Maria: A family that gets their...oscopies together stays together.

Nona: This is the funniest thing I've seen all day. You two sure know how to celebrate a milestone. Recover quickly.

Tina: The romance is real!

Transplant Team's blood test says no CMV virus, so that's a bullet dodged. Otherwise, I'd have to go back to a hospital bed.

That would've made me crankier than a yeti watching global warming melt his house.

(Meme) "An average of 22 people die each day waiting for a transplant. Every 10 minutes, someone is added to the national transplant waiting list."

7/5/19
Re-read the lab report on the new heart. It said at one point, "Gross photos were taken."

They certainly <u>were</u> gross.

Maria: Um...thanks for the warning?

Scott: Or did they mean that they took 144 of them?

Ana: That would have been bulk.

Sharon: Isn't that a ream, Scott?

A ream is 500 sheets of paper, people.

Scott: I don't ream-member.

Sharon: ♫ "Beautiful ream-er, wake unto me..."

Useless factoid: "Beautiful Dreamer" is the song that Terry Moore plays to control her giant ape in the 1949 film, 'Mighty Joe Young'. The Oscar-winning ape effects were done by Willis O'Brien, animator of 'King Kong,' and his young assistant, Ray Harryhausen.

Terry Moore was Mrs. Howard Hughes, which has to be the very definition of a mixed blessing. She's 86 and still acting.

Helen: Will that picture be in the book? It was unbelievable!!

Rebecca: Make sure to compare with a normal heart. My friend works for a group of cardiologists, and the perfusion tech looked at those pictures. He is a little surprised you are here.

Me: Yeah, I get that a lot.

75,000 words on the transplant memoir.

Mark: Vol. 1 and 2?

Me: *Heart Snark 2: The Legend of Curley's Gold.*

'The Biopsy Strikes Back.'

'The Bride of Frankenteacher.'

'Evil Dead 2' and 'Dawn of the Dead." (didn't even have to change those)

7/6/19
"My grandfather's work was...doodoo!" Yes, that line is actually in my heart transplant memoir. It does my heart good to say that.

Serge: Frau Blucher!

Matthew: *whinny*

Fun Fact: there's an urban legend that the horses whinny because 'blucher' is German for 'glue.' Not true, alas.

But...
General Blucher, defeater of Napoleon at Waterloo, did invent a popular military boot, which was made out of leather. So that would still make a horse nervous.

Garalt: Still deeper than "Baby Shark."

7/7/19
The new heart went in 3 months ago tonight. I marked this auspicious occasion by producing a stool sample and proudly

presenting it to the hospital lab like a kid showing his mommy the A+ on his book report.

Me: "It's not just my grandfather's work that was doodoo!"

Maria: Has it been that long? Wow...

Eileen: Ah, medicine. It never quite lets you loose, and yes, we are inordinately interested in that stuff.

Sharon: Splendid rendition of the power of poop!

Me: Told the hospital receptionist, "I'm here to give you some shit."

Maria: You are adorable.

'Adorkable', maybe.

Mark: Just how does one study for that test?

Lots of, um, cramming.

23 lab tests later, I'm negative for everything from salmonella to e. coli. I have pristine poop.

Tina: Well, now you have to tell us your secret.

I pay a hacker to change the results on the hospital computer.

Me: Most important: no infection from my now way-over-suppressed immune system.

So far, anyway.

Beverly: Thanks for sharing. The gauntlet is thrown...

Ana: What about the good strains of e coli? They only tested for bad ones?

Me: I am fond of Coca Coli.

Garalt: Did they screen for snark?

Yeah, they did. They're ordering a new machine as we speak. The old one threw itself out a window in despair.

Woke up with a mild groin strain yesterday. Hadn't done any running/biking to cause it, so I must've just slept in some bizarre position (not the first time).

Today it's a lot worse, but that's due to precisely the reason you filthy-minded monsters would think of first. #insertyourjokehere #JanetandIregretnothing

Hey, that teenaged heart doesn't mess around. "I play through pain like a boss!"

(Meme of 2 elderly Vikings with med bottles) "Face it, Sven. We're old. 'Pillage' doesn't mean what it used to mean."

7/8/19
At the movie theater watching Benedict Cumberbatch play Hamlet, in observance of my waking up from the transplant 3 months ago. Most appropriate lines: "Though hast cleft my heart in twain." "Oh, throw away the worser part."

In fact, throw the worser part into a burning dumpster, after driving a wooden stake through it (but make sure you send a sample off to the lab first).

7/9/19
Well, did a new blood test today and the low white cell count has barely budged, so they cancelled my Thursday endoscopy and dental cleaning, until I have an immune system that people don't laugh and point at.

No infection, though. My little guys are few, but studly.

Which reminds me of a line from 'A Midsummer Night's Dream': "Though she be but

little, she is fierce."

Me: In a week, the white cell count has jumped a whole .2. Same with the tacrolimus. So I have to get jabbed again next week to see if there's more progress. My white blood cells are 1/3 what they were the day before the transplant.

7/10/19
50km (31 miles) on the old today, including the climb of a short but nasty 13% hill. Had to stop to have my picture taken by some lady who adored the 'Old Fart Cycling Team' jersey.

Me: Haven't been able to do 30 miles in almost a year.

Hey, suicidal dumbass on the bike path riding with a straw hat. Why the hell aren't you wearing the helmet that's freaking ATTACHED TO YOUR BACKPACK???!!

Julie: Organ donor wannabe ?

Me: I don't want any of this guy's organs. He looked like a taste-tester at a Twinkie factory.

Me: But hey, at lest he was exercising, so points for that.

Janet's experiencing the splendiferous joy of colonoscopy prep tonight. She seems to feel that a PMS/menopause/leprosy cocktail would be preferable. #prayformysurvival

Got it all done, though. She was, um, flushed with pride.

Julia: I agree with her.

Sharon: True!! Pray they use sterilized equipment.

David: I suppose I should sympathize, but having been there, I'm laughing because I know how annoying it is.

Christine: While I agree with Janet, as Jim's sister pointed out, a colonoscopy allows the doc to find any cancerous lesions and snip them out before they become a bigger problem. Snip, you are cured!

Which is precisely what happened. All benign. She's good for 5 years.

Barbara: I like to think of the prep as "spring cleaning."

Maria: This is one of my "landed on the Moon" complaints. We landed a man on the moon but we cannot separate certain medical procedures from medieval torture.

Jim: Well, actually (in his best mansplaining voice): There is a service my son (who has these regularly) has pondered. You arrive a few hours earlier for the event. No prep needed. Before the actual event, they... clean you out. Kinda like hooking up a vacuum hose. He hasn't done it, but it's been tempting...

One imagines a bicycle pump and garden hose...

Janet: I agree with Maria. This is torture. Waking up at 4am to down another bottle of nuclear colon cleanser, after a week without food of any value and a day of just liquids, is making me feel woozy and nauseous. I came close to upchucking the second dose, but willed myself to keep down that $104 of medicine.

Garalt: Oh, don't, they're doing that to me, too, soon. Here's hoping it all goes well.

Janet: The procedure itself is nothing compared to a week's worth of prep. 6 days of only foods with no color or more than 1 gram of fiber, no seeds, skins, pulp, no dyes, spices, only over-cooked veggies, potatoes, pasta, white rice, white bread, vanilla pudding and crackers, and if you eat meat, only white chicken. The last day is just clear liquid and then the doses of colon cleanser. Can't go more than a few feet away from the bathroom. As a general rule, we avoid white bread and most of those foods because they aren't good for you. By day 5 I lost all appetite and stopped eating anyway. Good way to lose weight, though. I wonder how we survived in the 50's eating that stuff all the time. Remember all the PB&J sandwiches on Wonder Bread? Ugh.

Janet: What ever happened to enemas or colonics? I've seen *The Road to Wellville* **(link # 10)**. They used to do them. 15 gallons of yoghurt.

Matthew Broderick: "Oh, no, no, I can't eat fifteen gallons of yoghurt."
Anthony Hopkins: "Oh, it's not going in **that** *end, Mr. Lightbody."*

The 'Road to Wellville' (from T.C. Boyle's book) is one weird and highly overstaffed flick (Hopkins, Broderick, John Cusack, Bridget Fonda, etc.). John Harvey Kellogg (yes, the corn flakes family) ran a health/wellness sanitarium in the late 1800's that employed some way out of the (cereal)box methods (like those yoghurt enemas). Seems he was obsessed with the lower half of one's body and all of the goings-on there.

"An erection is a flagpole on your grave!" (I bet this made Mrs. Kellogg really happy)

"One should never, ever, interrupt one's desire to defecate. I have inquired at the zoos as to the daily bowel evacuations of primates. At the end of an average day, their cages are filled with a veritable mountain of natural health."

"My own stools, sir, are gigantic and have no more odor than a hot biscuit."

7/11/19
In the hospital (aka 'The House of Pain', a la *The Island of Lost Souls;* link #11) waiting room for Janet's colonoscopy. 2 days of prep for a 15-minute procedure, according to the tech who came to take her back. I offered to trade her medical issues, but no (though I swear she gave it some thought).

Yeah, I just ordered an Impossible Burger…with bacon. That's how I roll.

Cameron: We call that a 'hypocrite burger.'

Dave: Schrodinger's Quarter Pounder.

Cynthia: You're even eating like a 19-year-old?

7/12/19
17th anniversary today. Not sure what that makes this. It's not silver or gold. Polyethylene, maybe.

Liana: Plastic containers is the 17th. By now you probably have an entire matching set of every size, shape, and capacity. Of course, none of the lids you also have match any of the containers, but you've got 'em.

Harriet: 17 is a Prime number. Something from Amazon Prime?

So is 61. Clearly, I'm in my prime. Oh, and Jeff Bezos, you now owe me money for the ad.

The nurse said that Janet was a lightweight, anesthesia-wise. Hardly a surprise. She can barely handle half a bottle of Guinness stout. They said the same about me. Just another warm and fuzzy reason for our marital bliss.

(Janet) I seem to have missed that part of the red-haired gene, thankfully.

Me: (slurring words badly) "Bartender! Another round of Fentanyl for my friends!"

Maria: When Gerry had his knee surgery couple of months ago, he came out of the anesthesia so violently, they had to summon a sturdy nurse named Matt to subdue him while another nurse stuck him with another tranquilizer.

This is why they need automated veterinary dart guns installed up in the corners of each room.

School isn't for a month yet, but the teacher nightmares have started. Wandering around the newly constructed part of the school, trying to find the virginal classroom they're building for me as we speak, getting totally lost. At least the 'naked and don't know anything about your subject' part hasn't begun yet.

Me: I'm guessing that right now it wouldn't be the naked part that would horrify people as much as the Frankenstein part.

Rebecca: I just had one where I had to teach a class but had not prepped. Nobody would tell me where and what time. It does not stop after you are retired

Julie: Perhaps your heart isn't in it yet.

Maria: Make sure you are nice to the virginal classroom. It hadn't seen much of the world yet. This experience will mean everything.

Me: I'll be gentle. Flowers and dinner first, then the furniture gets rammed in.

We went to Sherpa's in Boulder for lunch. (photos 83, 84)

That's a restaurant owned by actual Nepalese sherpas. The owner has climbed Everest a gazillion times.

Rebecca: Wow, both of you great. Being young at heart agrees with you.

Kelly: You look really good with good color in your face.

Me: Yeah, well, green is a color.

7/13/19
Managed a whole 3 chin-ups today. Believe it or not, that's actually progress.

A year or so ago I could do almost 20.

Samantha: I couldn't even do at that my peak of health so…good job!

Chris: Chin up, soldier!

Just jogged 200 steps, which sounds lame but I haven't been able to run that far since last fall, with the old horror-heart.

Which I clearly should not have been doing back then.

10 pushups with my resurrected sternum.

(Meme) "Tradition is just peer pressure from dead people."

7/14/19
Because I didn't already have enough Shakespeare tchotchkes in my life. (photo 85)

7/15/19
Just managed to run 250 steps (1/6 mile) 3 times at 10:00/mile pace. Then sprinted 100 meters twice at a sub-6:00 pace. No heart failure, stroke, or pulled muscles. #advancingrapidlynow

It's Janet's birthday, so in my never-ending quest to demonstrate my romantic bona fides to the men of America, we're off to buy toilet paper.

Yeah, I'm Prince Charmin.

Ali: Curiously, I ordered two 9 roll packs earlier. Happy birthday, Janet.

Me: Great minds think alike.

Serge: L'amour, toujours l'amour!

Liana: She'll be thrilled. Did you wrap them with paper and ribbon?

Me: Gold foil, of course.

Tina: You have out-done yourself this year, Terry! Do you have an available brother? I'm green with envy!

Me: I was green a few weeks ago, but envy had little to do with it.

Me: One brother, utterly unlike me (to be fair I'M the weird one), married for 30+ years.

Rose: It's not true love if it isn't two-ply...

JP: Wow. My husband just takes me to the landfill. He's gonna have to step up his game!

Me: We DID go to a swanky Italian restaurant first.

Jami: But how was THEIR toilet paper?

Me: Like a fine gelato.

Mark: Can always get the expensive brand.

Me: Favorite all-time movie line: "I love to curse in French. It's like wiping your ass with silk." (one of the *Matrix* flicks)

This book manuscript is 300 pages already.

Continuing our toilet paper theme...

"Have you ever considered being a phlebotomist?"

"No, but I suppose I could take a stab at it." (rim shot)

"Thank you, thank you! It's great to be back on 'Comedians in Cars Getting Heckled.'

Me: Don't any of you needle me about my puns.

Me: I'm going to bleed this topic for all of its humor.

Me: I'm vein about my punning ability.

Me: My favorite Christmas carol is "The Holly and the IV."

Me: We can have a phlebotomy pun-off: a sort of competition, a single-elimination tourniquet, if you will.

Scott: Okay, we get the point.

Me: Sorry, I'm going to stick to it.

Scott: OK, give it a shot.

Liana: These puns just aren't my type.

Scott: O, be positive.

Liana: Are you trying to make my comment look like A negative? That's pretty rare.

Scott: And with that, A-B, A-B, A-B, that's all, folks!

Me: There's an awful 'clot' of puns here…emphasis on 'awful.'

7/16/19
This is Day 100 with the new heart.
In honor of the occasion, I went to the hospital for another blood test and Janet ordered titanium kitchen strainers. #settingthebarhigh

Yeah, we have a strained relationship.

It occurs to me that I've only had 5 real surgical procedures, not counting catheters into veins for lookie-loos. Hernia repair as a baby, a tonsillectomy in 1967, an appendectomy in 2013, pacemaker, and this year's heart transplant. So nearly every surgical event involves cutting stuff out and throwing it away.

Actually, 6 procedures, if you count that unfortunate willie-snipping in infancy.

Pretty sure they took too much off on that last one.

Got a letter from the Neptune Society today, about cremation. Hopefully they don't know something I don't. And shouldn't it really be the Vulcan Society?

Me: Vulcan Society motto: "Face it, you aren't going to live long and prosper."

Veronica: They have an underwater garden with statues somewhere.

Me: Key Biscayne, Florida. They'll turn you into concrete and make you part of a dive site.

That'll cement your reputation after you're gone.

7/17/19
(Cartoon: Mom sewing Frankenstein monster on kitchen table for 2 boys: "Next time you boys wait till the last minute to ask me for help with a school project, you're on your own.") They actually did this to me late on a Sunday night. It <u>was</u> a teaching hospital.

Despite giving 4 vials of blood for tests yesterday, the Transplant Team made me go back today for more. My white blood cells are practically non-existent, thanks to the rejection meds, so they're taking me off of the Valcyte (for CMV virus prevention), as it nukes white cells. But they want a CMV test as a baseline. #heyit'sonlyblood

Me: The hospital receptionist recognizes me on sight now and just waves me through.

Maria: You know...somewhere there is like small town-style water tower filled with your blood. It all has to go somewhere, and I haven't heard of any major chemical spills lately, so it has to be how they store it.

That would explain why we have to filter the water at our house.

It's true, I have trouble being serious about my near-fatal medical

issues. I have...snarkoidosis.

Jami: How long have you been waiting to bless us with that one?

7/18/19
Managed to run a whole mile today, in small chunks. Can now run a quarter-mile at a 10:00/mile pace before having to stop and suck air for a minute. Extending the running distance and cutting the rest time bit by bit. Some day this new heart will be trained to the level of the old one, or as close as I can get it). It's only been 3 months since it went in. I have an organ donors 'race' this Sunday, which I'll clearly be walking. Except for the last ¼-mile, so I can heroically run across the finish line where the cameras will be.

Liana: Oh. I was wondering...I mean, do you really WANT the organs of those who collapse?

I think you've been misunderstanding how we get organs. You might want to sit down for this one...

The most recent blood test didn't change much. The tacrolimus (rejection med) level did go up, from 8.8 to 10.0. Okay, in the safe zone, but not quite where they want it (12-13). The white blood cell count actually went **DOWN** a tiny fraction. It's at 2.2 and should really be no lower than 4, 3 at the worst, for a transplant patient. That makes me neutropenic (sounds like somebody the Avengers have to defend Earth from). Had to get a separate test yesterday for a baseline CMV level, since they'll have to closely monitor it in lieu of having the med suppress it. Result was completely negative, so that's good. If the count isn't up by the 30th, they won't be able to do my next biopsy the next day. #andthepageantcontinues

My white cells just had a Viking funeral...

7/19/19
Because America demanded this. (photos 86, 87)

Donna: And by 'America' you mean...?

I mean I was bored, needed a Facebook post for today, and happened to be wearing that shirt.

Jeanne: When one of the kids asks my father how he got the big scar on his chest, he tells them he ate a roll of toilet paper and they had to operate to get it out.

Barbara: They'll fade over time. I had 31 staples from sternums to waistline. Scar is still there, of course, but it's lighter. Gastro-tube scar is barely visible.

15 easy miles on the bike today, since I have a 5K 'race' on Sunday. Well, it would've been easy if I hadn't done all of that running in the heat yesterday.

Me: Got to love-up an adorable basset hound puppy on the bike path. #win

(meme) "Stop naming hospitals after dead people. Give us some hope! Where's the Keith Richards Memorial Hospital?"

Just ran the numbers and, at current prescribed levels, I'll take almost 10,000 med doses in a year.

Marion: Serious question: How does this work with your digestion and what about interactions? (I'm thinking of how difficult it can be to manage even the few prescriptions and supplements I take, and how many medications I dread taking because of side effects like nausea, upset stomach etc.).

Me: It utterly sucked at first, but now things have settled down. Not sure if that's my system getting used to all of that stuff or what.

Robin: You could probably replace all that bad shit with 365 doses of good cannabis.

I could. They'd block the rejection meds and I'd croak, but I'd be giggling when I went.

"Dude! Look! We're flatlinin'! Hand me that bag of Doritos. And don't Bogart the inspirometer."

7/20/19
2 ½ weeks till I'm back in the classroom...assuming I have enough immune system by then that they'll let me be around 171 germy urchins.

Rebecca: With no white cells, I doubt it. I think I caught everything going around when I taught.

I'll just get 171 sets of masks and gloves. Then I'll build a great big beautiful wall around my desk and get the district to pay for it.

7/21/19
At the 20th annual Donor Dash run/all event. 6500 participants, plus their dogs in tutus.

In my case, it'll be more of a Donor Stumble and Stagger. (88)

Sarah: You look thrilled.

Ana: I say he looks...dashing.

Rebecca: Looking good, and your color gets better every picture.

Soon I'll be up to the shade of an actual, living person.

Yeah...this happened.

5K/3.1 miles. Ran 2/3 of it, in 250-step chunks.

Heart transplant was 105 days ago. (photo 89)

Me: Got to love up on a total stranger's basset hound again.

Maria: Your dog will want to know where you've been, what you've been doing, and which strange basset hound you've been doing it with.

I'm such a belly-rub slut.

Rebecca: Congrats, that's more than I can do.

Glenna: You are an inspiration.

Fiona: You actually are far too fit for your own good...stop it immediately!

Our new sphygmomanometer (blood pressure thingie) is a hoot. It talks to you. A lady voice tells you what to do to get started, then cheesy elevator music plays while it's working, and she comes back to read out your numbers and say whether it's normal or not, according to the World Health Organization.

Me: I hope she doesn't refuse to open the pod bay doors.

(Janet) Can't say that I care for it. I don't like electronic devices that mindlessly talk to you.

Well, this is just great. The FDA put out a notice that there's a nationwide shortage of tacrolimus, my main anti-rejection med. Good thing I just got refilled.

How many flippin' people are getting transplants this month??? Is there a big ½-off sale? 'Die one, get one free?'

7/23/19
Janet finally got new glasses today, after months of near blindness because they kept changing her blood pressure meds and thus messing with her eyes. This is important because when she had to drive me to the ER on the night of March 30, I literally had to describe the road to her while I was in ventricular tachycardia. It's an utter miracle that I lived to get the heart transplant.

Need a couple of white canes for our fenders...or a seeing-eye greyhound.

Maria: You guys are NOT boring — that's for damn sure.

Today's creepy adventure: Janet had me try on her long-deceased mom's glasses and I could see out of them just as perfectly as with my new ones I got last fall.

Maria: I am sure there is a horror story in there somewhere.

Janet: Of course, no mention of the fact that after seeing husband get shocked and revived and bundled up to go in the ambulance to Anshutz, I had to drive myself home blind at 12am. Took me longer to get out of the maze that is the parking lot than it took to go home.

Adding a half/serious/half snarky medical terms glossary to the heart transplant memoir. There are nearly 100 of the suckers.

7/25/19
Making up medical terms funny is harder than it sounds. This may take a while.

Me: 'Allograft: a transplant of tissue/organ from someone who isn't you; not to be confused with graft, which is stealing from someone who isn't you.'

Just a thought. Blood vessels...are there Crips vessels, too?
Do they sail the Red Sea and the Blue Nile?

Me: And is that tiny submarine in *Fantastic Voyage* also a blood vessel?

Michael: That faint rumble you heard was me groaning at this from a thousand miles away.

Me: Then my work here is done.

7/26/19
37 medical bills came into the iPad at 1 a.m. The pings sounded like a drunk pounding on a hotel bell. Good thing we've reached our out-of-pocket max for the year.

Mandy: What does the out-of-pocket thing mean?

Me: After we've paid $4000, the insurance pays the rest until the end of the year. In our case, close to $2 million.

Mandy: Yikes!

Current bill for all of this heart transplant stuff: $1,905,541.45.

Me: This is the retail price. That's not what the insurance company paid, of course. They cut a deal with the hospital for less than $500,000. A deal I would absolutely NOT get if I was paying cash.

Theresa: They can write off a majority of it, believe it or not.

Alaena: So, kinda like the Kohls retail system of pricing? We were just in the mall and that crap drives me nuts. Especially since one of the high-end stores was closing. Saw a little sweater in the window I just loved. 40% lowest ticketed. Retail on this sweater was $820. Lowest marked price was $280. Even at 40% off that, there is no way in hell. I'm sad, I liked it.

I liked my old heart, too…until it tried to murder me.
Pretty sure they tossed it into the bargain bin.

Cerene: Average weight of a human heart: 310g.
Current value of 1g of gold: $45.67.
That means they've charged the price for over 131 'hearts of gold'.

Me: My weight in gold is around $3.4 million. Not far to go.

Fiona: Dear god! Just had a quick check on the actual costs on the NHS of a heart transplant. £40,000 for the op plus £60,000 in post op care and immunosuppressant drugs…that figure includes staffing costs! There's something very, very wrong going on there.

Shaindel: Please remember that there are people who are allowed to die because they are not considered financially viable for transplant. You are incredibly privileged.

Me: Absolutely true, alas. *And enraging.*

Karen: So glad I live in Canada. The bill for my husband's open-heart surgery was $0.

Tara: Wow! That's a LOT. I'm in the hole $4200 for going to a hospital without insurance, because I couldn't keep fluids down. Definitely think I should have risked death instead, but here we are.

Toni: Tara, heed my advice. They triple charge people without insurance because there are no insurance execs to whittle down the price. I was able to get 20 -30% off by haggling. I was lucky enough to see a news blurb about it, just before my son went in. Good luck and hope you're all better!

Tara: Thanks. I tried, and they wouldn't haggle unless I had a lot of money (to pay it off outright). I'm wondering if there is a professional I could hire to do that (?). I'm pretty bad at that myself. Seems like unless I have thousands ready to fork over, they're not interested in haggling. Did you have a lot of $ on hand when you haggled?

Toni: Nope. Once they get your money, it's never coming back. Small monthly payments. You need time to make all those calls, however. I almost called an ambulance for my son (he lives in Santa Monica), but I was quoted 4 grand for that. He called Uber instead. Granted he had a 106 degree fever at the time, so it wasn't easy. You just need to open up to a kind sounding person at the various offices. They know they over-charge, so often 20% off is what they're expecting.

Toni: It's really horrible. They truly do cheat the uninsured. I told each agent about what I'd heard on the news about the 300% increase. They're only allowed to help so much, but sometimes it's worth the haggling. Frankly, they probably only do about $500 worth of work for the $4 grand you pay out. Now, that I've hijacked Terry's thread, let me just say Terry, OUCH!!!

Janet: They do a thorough evaluation to determine if you are a candidate for a transplant, insurance and financial status being a big part of it. If we hadn't sold our duplex last year, we wouldn't have had the $4000 on hand for the out of pocket. Plus, the surgery was done at the perfect time so that Terry had enough accumulated time off to cover all but 5 days of the school year. They evaluate a patient's ability to follow the medication schedule and the instructions, too, which almost require a college education. Plus, a support system which, without our daughter and a friend who loves our basset hound, would have been very difficult. All the stars lined up and Terry is here because of it. His old heart was not going to keep him going much longer and even the experts were surprised at how bad it was, so he was very lucky.

Fiona: While I am eternally grateful the stars aligned and Mr. Snarkypants is still with us, I am still utterly horrified by any medical system that requires insurance agents and financiers to decide whether it is worth saving someone. It seems to me to be the complete opposite to the Hippocratic Oath all doctors sign to 'do no harm'. And that ' All life is sacred'. Even more so in a so-called civilized society. I guess I knew this intellectually but this is the first time I've seen evidence from someone I actually know. And I find it horrifying and appalling and utterly inhuman. For people to panic over whether they can afford an ambulance, or to know things would have worked out very differently for you guys if the situation had been a little different.... I'm glad it wasn't. But this is not a civilized way to behave as a country. I have no idea how the US ended up this way.

We ended up this way because one political party seems to think that helping people is some sort of 'Communist plot.' That's really how they put it.

Maria: We need to get single payer, Medicare for All, something. That is ridiculous. This is why so many people choose to go to Thailand for operations. I would if I needed something important.

7/27/19
21 miles on the bike and a chiropractic adjustment. Nap time.

*See? I **am** well-adjusted!*

7/29/19
I guess 4 miles and 9000 steps is enough before 10 a.m. Ran most of the middle 2 miles, 300 steps at a time with a 100-step walk in between.

Me: 13,000 steps for the day.

Weird Thing of the Day: Amazon actually has an Organ Transplant bestsellers list.

When this book dropped on Kindle, it was the #1 New Release in cardiology. #2 was 'Guidewire and Catheter Skills for Endovascular Surgery.'

7/30/19
Nothing more fun than literally jumping out of bed to go get blood drawn at the hospital. But at least my white blood cell count is up, too.

7/31/19
Up at 4 a.m. so we can check in at Anschutz at 6 a.m. for a biopsy. #thefunneverstops

Maria: Is it that time of the month again?

Julie: I had a double take moment there. I thought you wrote 'Auschwitz.'

It occurs to me that going back over all of the transplant FB posts for the book and adding jokes is just me doing Mystery Science Theatre to myself.

Kathryn: ^ This post also qualifies as book fodder.

Neck aches from the biopsy. Considering he was Dr. Swat, I shouldn't be surprised.

Me: I had a literal Swat Team working on me today.

Ana: Buffy's vet is Dr. Depaw. The world is full of coincidences and puns.

Me: I had a dentist named Toothaker.

And I'm going to keep mentioning it until somebody laughs.

Ana: And just read a friend's post and we have a Dr. Wheezer as a pulmonologist.

Today's blood tests show mostly the same as yesterday's. They aren't happy with my immune system and the kidney stress isn't anything to write home about, either. Took me off my unnecessary blood pressure meds to help fix the latter.

Maria: Well...considering how many meds you are on it's no surprise your kidneys and liver are struggling. Maybe you should have one of my radioactive kidneys, after all.

Rebecca: Are you sure you do not need the blood pressure meds with school starting Tuesday?

Me: Hey, I don't get high blood pressure, I CAUSE it.

When I went off the BP meds, there was literally no difference in the readings.

Have to take Boniva now, since the meds tend to wreck your bones. Only once a month, so you know it's ass-kickingly potent and probably burns a hole through you. #bone-appetit

Me: Same counter-intuitive possible side effects: femur fractures and osteonecrosis (bone death) of the jaw.

Rebecca: I get shots every six months.

Me: I DO shots every 6 months.

It turned out to not be much of a problem, at least for the first dose.

The transplant cardiologist couldn't get his seat to stay up where he wanted it today, so I asked him if he was having trouble with his stool sample.

Headline: 'Johns Hopkins performs world's first total penis transplant.' (link #12)

I hope it wasn't from a living donor.

Me: And why would you do a less-than-total penis transplant? What is that anyway, surgeons working for, um, tips?

The earlier penis transplants...petered-out before the end.

At the blood draw today, we met a guy who'd had a kidney transplant, fellow of color, very outgoing and garrulous. From Baltimore. He'd spent 12 years in jail in his youth, and turned himself around when he saw that Ben Carson had done some amazing surgical feat. "I never knew people who looked like me could do that." He set some sort of record on the college entrance exam. This being America, the white proctor thought he'd cheated and made him retake it while being stared at. Same result. They enrolled him instantly, to their credit.

He ended up working for 30 years as a surgical assistant...for heart transplants.

Me: Said he wrote a memoir. Haven't found it yet.

Me: He had to sell drugs to pay for his transportation to school. The cop who arrested him every week eventually gave him the $ instead.

Washing hands in the Cardiology bathroom today and I stepped on something solid. I cursed the incompetent custodial staff and looked to see what it was. Somebody had dropped a wedding ring. I picked it up with my left hand and noticed who exactly it belonged to. #slipperyfingers

The Precious was seeking its master…Janet was only 30 feet away.

8/1/19
All 3 grandkids inbound today, so you know what that means: sterilizing the whole house when they leave like it's an Ebola zone. #transplantproblems

Evaluating HEPA filters for my classroom. Hoping they filter out all sounds from troublesome students, too. #aguycanhope

4 chin-ups/20 push-ups. Really making impressive progress on this whole post-transplant upper-body strength thing.

But hey, 4/20, baby!

Maria: I can't do a chin-up if you paid me.

Me: In the army I could do close to 100 push-ups, 80+ sit-ups, 15 chin-ups, and run 2 miles in 10 minutes, plus pass the Army Ranger swim test in full uniform/weapon. #badassbackintheday

Maria: I can do a four-hour Zumba marathon. Does that count?

8/2/19
Yeah, I had to use a Lysol wipe to sanitize my bottle of hand sanitizer. #transplantgiggles

Multiple degrees in Theatre, Fine Arts, and Fashion Design between us, and we're off to see that classic of introspective cinema, *Hobbs and Shaw.*

8/3/19
This is the instruction/warning/info sheet that came with my ONE osteoporosis pill today. It's nearly 2 feet across, tiny print, double-sided. (photo 90)

Scott: Looks like a CVS receipt!

Cardio-vascular silliness? Can't visualize sarcoidosis? Cardio-death's Very Shitty?

Sean: Make the print 12 pt. and you can use it as the second volume of your transplant saga.

Cal: What happens if you don't read it? I never follow instructions since I was a kid. Just go with the gut and do it.

Your face melts off like the Nazis in 'Raiders of the Lost Ark.'

Helen: Is it in several languages like stuff from IKEA?!

Me: Nope.

Came with an Allen wrench, though. That scares me.

Randall: I had a doc that said don't ever read those things. They'll scare you.

Jeri: I think if you submit that, you can get a PhD.

Karen: Decoupage it to a table, it's very interesting.

Carol: What is the name of the med, with instructions like that?

Me: Boniva.

Not to be confused with Bovina, goddess of dairy farmers.

8/4/19
25 miles on the bike. That's plenty. It's already pushing 90 degrees. Any farther and I'd be pushing the bike. Archie McThump-Thump

got up to 165 bpm on the hill. He needs a nap.

Me: 10th ride since the heart transplant. About 200 miles total.

(cartoon of an alien singing on stage) 'Aria 51.'

'Madame Butterflying Saucer.'

Janet always says that I'm the sickest healthy person ever. Here's a breakdown from top to bottom:

**no hair
autism
cataracts
myopia
astigmatism
tinnitus
deviated septum
hypothyroid
reflux
dead heart**

*And I'm **still** healthier than most of the population.*

**8/5/19
Just bought so many cleaning/sanitizing supplies at Sam's Club that they probably think we're serial killers scrubbing a crime scene.**

Maria: Let them. Maybe next time they'll cut you a better deal.

Rebecca: Did you buy the large black trash bags and duck tape?

Me: Didn't want to be too obvious. We aren't amateurs.

New total for all of this heart stuff: $1,946,965.37.

$1.98 million as of publication.

8/6/19
First day back at school and the district is trying to kill me already by putting me in a meeting cheek-by-jowl with 1500 germy people. #anotherdaywithnoimmunesystem

Me: May have to fake cardiac distress and flee.

Me: The @#$! noise isn't helping my autistic sensitivity, either.

Mark: Remember to take your giant plastic bubble next time.

Scott: Ugh...I remember days like this...sends chills of anxiety and stress down my spine. Run, Terry, run from all of it!

Me: I'm trapped. The heart can't do that yet.

Me: Sitting on the aisle, so one side would be safe, and the guy next to me moved over to leave an empty seat to help me out. He's a science teacher.

Maria: I don't suppose it's in the budget to equip you with a hazmat suit?

I needed a garden sprayer full of Purell.

Told to be here at 7:45 for this vitally important teacher mob. It's now 8:30 and nothing has happened yet. If you're going to waste my time, at least alert me to the fact.

Me: I wonder what 'cutting-edge teaching technique' we have to focus on this year. No doubt it will just be a renamed version of something that was invented in 1887.

Me: Superintendent did his thing and sprung us 30 minutes early. And THAT'S why he was Superintendent of the Year.

35 boxes picked up and opened in the new classroom, which is, of

course, the closest new thing to the main office, so I'll be on the freaking 'VIP tour' showing off the pretty and expensive toy. They may regret that. #nosocialskills #atleastthebathroomisclose (photo 91)

Erin: Do you really have a room with no windows? It really looks like there are zero windows. That is so not healthy.

Me: 2 solar tubes, which is more than I've had for the 15 years prior. #notthesamething

Me: Why, no, the air conditioning isn't working. Thank you for asking.

And, of course, the A/C came on as I was leaving.

We all got swanky $40 Nike polo shirts with the school logo. Your tax dollars at work.

Sitting here sweating my life away, waiting for this wretched MacBook update to load. Says 35 minutes to go.

It was as bad as the Box in 'Cool Hand Luke.' "What we have here is a failure to refrigerate."

8/7/19

4 months ago to the minute they were wheeling me into surgery prep for the heart transplant. Now I'm setting up my classroom for the students I'll have next Wednesday.

Judith: It's been a textbook recovery.

Russell: You're insane.

Me: Already established. Anything else?

8/8/19
Not sure my transplant team would be jumping for joy at me hauling a big-ass table, over 4 feet across, from my old room to the new, or lugging 36 boxes of mostly books, in no air conditioning. #toolateit'sdone

Sarah: Let's be real. Your transplant team would not be happy if they knew half the crap you have done since the surgery.

Dave: Maybe draft a crew next time and bribe them with pizza.

Janet: Make sure the school gets the pros to move the shelves. Of course, they promise help that never comes but keep nagging them. Getting help is always a challenge.

That's what happened, eventually.

Maria: I am surprised your transplant team doesn't have you considered in some sort of transplant jail.

"The castle doesn't stand that can hold me. Post your guards!" – Anthony Hopkins, 'The Lion in Winter.'

8/9/19
Think about it. (photo 92)

Me: I'm sure I'll be peppered with groans.

Rebecca: I feel for Janet having to live with the puns.

Me: 'Having to live' with? Don't you mean 'GETTING to live' with?

Mark: Yeah, it's corny.

Me: That's okay, I'm a seasoned pro.

Me: It's a powerful pun.

Mark: They're both conductive in water.

Stephanie: This took me ages because my mind immediately went in a sexual direction! But damn it if I could find a sexual pun!

Me: "She caught Himalayan her sister."

Me: "But she knew that if she killed him, the judge would throw her into a Duracell for life."

Colorado humor:

Dude: "Doc, I have joint pain."
Doctor: "That's because you're smoking the wrong end."

8/10/19
Great. Now Amazon's sending me e-mails suggesting transplant books I might be interested in. The only one I want is the one I just wrote.

8/11/19
From a goofy list of such jokes: *Irish Heart Surgery*, by Angie O'Plasty.

Mark: They forgot *Holes in the Mattress* by Mister Completely, and *Under the Bleachers* by Seymour Butts, and *Working at the Gas Station* by Phil R. Up.

Me: *Getting Old Sucks* by I. P. Knightly.

Mark: *The Things in the Bottles*, co-written by Kay O' Pectate, Anna Sinn, Al K. Seltzer, Ty Lenol, Gerry Tol, and Auntie Histamine.

(Headline) "Bride walked down aisle by man with her father's heart." (link #13)

Jim: Gosh-darn onion ninjas...

8/12/19
I have TWO HUNDRED students this year. WTF???
SO glad I moved heaven and earth to stay alive.

Janet: And I'm sure you will impress upon every one of the kids that they
are very lucky to have you alive, making the sacrifice to teach them.

Scott: "I had the choice between angels and you guys, and I picked you.
Remember that."

*"Remember, I've already been gutted like a fish by masked men with knives and saws.
So sit the hell down and do your assignment."*

**(Headline) "World's First 3D Printed Hearts and Functional Beating
Hearts Grown From Stem Cells." (link #14)**

Do those penis-transplant people know about this?

8/13/19
The first Shakespeare in the Park posters are up! (photo 93)

A theatre group in Dublin is using images of me as Shakespeare on their posters.
***That'll** put butts in the seats.*

Me: Damn, I look good in brocade.

Maria: Um... Duh!

**REALLY glad this first day of school was freshmen only (I don't
teach those urchins), because otherwise the students would've been
exposed to the charming sight of me curled up in a corner literally
crying from transplant-med reflux. Felt like an actual heart attack.
Reminder: stomach acid is stronger than battery acid and will eat
through metal. You make a liter and a half of it every day.
#we'reallpoisonfactories**

Fiona: Flipping heck mate! Are you sure you're good to be back at work yet? I know you're a superhuman and all...but please put you first!

Me: Haven't had one of those that bad in 3 months. Hardly ever have reflux at all anymore.

Fiona: Mayhap returning to work adds stress??? Reflux in general is a known stress symptom. Just saying, hun. Are you sure you're ready? Do NOT want to lose you, too. Xxxx

Compared to recent events, school no longer has any ability to deliver stress.

Me: No, it goes away eventually. This one was only super-bad for about 30 minutes. The rest of the hour+ was just ordinary esophageal misery.

Janet: The reflux has been a problem all along, even before the transplant, but seems to be seasonal also. It was bad in the spring, right after the transplant, and not so frequent all summer. New school year jitters, probably, and breathing all the dust from construction. Coming up with a way to get through bouts of it while teaching is going to be a challenge. Not working would mean no insurance for doctors and meds. Retiring early and supplementing income with online teaching to pay for insurance might be necessary, but we'll have to see how it goes.

8/14/19
Proof that I lived to teach again. (photo 94)

Me: Well, I CALL it teaching.

M Cid: I thought you only taught Lamaze.

Yeah. I use a catcher's mitt when I'm down there encouraging the mother.

Ana: That's a weird setup, the kids have to turn their heads to look at the screen? At least you don't have to look them in the eye.

Me: Oh, believe me, they turn their heads plenty anyway.

Tina: But, first…did you show them your scar? That would put the fear of Gawd in them!

Me: Just the top part. I DID show them the old dead heart.

Overjoyed at my new merino wool socks.
Yeah, it's a sheep thrill.

Me: Sorry…it had to be said.

Me: They were expensive. I may have been fleeced.

Me: These jokes are baaad.

Me: What do Marines call sheep? War brides.

Julie: With a joke that bad you should sheepishly hang your head.

Mark: I always knew you were a wolf in sheep's clothing.

Me: I'm a SHEEP in sheep's clothing, alas.

Fiona: They were clearly not a baaaaargain!

8/15/19
Having a school assembly tomorrow. They told me to write my own introduction, so:

"Mark Twain said, 'The reports of my death are greatly exaggerated.' Mr. Kroenung was only MOSTLY dead. He and his new heart are having fun storming the castle."

UPDATE: Well, that was a waste of wit. All they did was have us walk across the gym as a group while the students cheered ironically.

Janet: Are you going to wear one of your heart T-shirts?

Scott: "We are glad to report that, contrary to years of student evaluations, Mr. Kroenung is not heartless. We know because we've seen it firsthand."

Yeah, but it looked like Scrooge's heart.

Jim: "I was recently cast as the Tin Man in a production of *Wizard of Oz.* Since I am so completely a method actor, they had to give me a new heart after the show closed."

♬ *"When a man's an empty kettle…"*

Elise: Will they get it?

Me: Without a doubt. This is a nerdy school.

Jim: You can do the Yorick speech with your squeezy heart.

Me: The Ghost speech would be even better.

Yeah, I'm showing photos of my old dead heart to students on the first day. Have to establish my dominance early.

Helen: I can honestly say it is the most amazing thing I have ever seen. I show it to people who moan about their problems....

Alaena: It is actually kinda cool.

Tina: Way to establish who calling the shots. Next, will you show your scar?

Me: Well, the top part, anyway. Disrobing in class would be...problematic.

Chris: Just like the silverback gorillas do it.

8/16/19
So somebody above my pay grade dismissed the assembly 30 minutes early and I'm now expected to come up with something for this class to do for TWO FREAKING HOURS!!

Jim: Give students famous Shakespeare passages, and ask them to rewrite into modern language.

Dave Dahl's example: Romeo's balcony speech.
Original: "But soft, what light through yonder window breaks?"
Modern: "Damn! That bitch is fine!"

Jim: Or — loose the chaos on the administrators. Create a scavenger hunt. Give all students all-access multi-passes to go anywhere. Ensure that many items require exploration of the administrative offices.

Maria: I love this! Better yet — a heart transplant-themed scavenger hunt. Overlay the map of the school with the anatomy chart of a human body, and have the students find all the locations involved in the transplant life support.

Jim: Lungs overlay the HVAC system. Urinary and/or circulatory system overlays the plumbing. But…question — are the administrative offices overlaid by the cranial region, or the other end?

Scott: Retire.

I took his sage advice 2 years later. Now I never know what day of the week it is.

Me: I did what I had planned and then let them play on their phones. Sue me. #electronicpedogogy

Karen: Read excerpts from your manuscript.

Me: "It was a dark and stormy night...when they yanked my beating heart out."

Marisa: I keep reading "pay grade" as gay parade.

That would at least enliven the proceedings with fabulousness.

And, as I predicted with 100% certainty, my classroom air conditioning came on just in time for the last class of the steamy week.

(cartoon) "Tragic, really. He died because no one knew his blood type. I'll never forget the last inspirational words he whispered to me: 'Be positive.'"

(meme) Me, young and naïve: 'I hope something good happens.'

Me, now: 'I hope that whatever bad thing happens is at least funny.'

Hey, I'm doing my part on the 'funny disaster' train.

8/17/19
50 km (31 miles) on the bike again. Climbed a series of short, punchy hills at gradients of 5% to 13%. I doubt that those had ANYTHING to do with my subsequent leg cramps.

Maria: Mutant.

That's MISTER Mutant to you.

(seen on Twitter someplace) "Saying that teachers only work 7 a.m.-3 p.m. 10 months a year is like saying that Tom Brady only works a few Sundays a year."

(cartoon of doctor speaking while nurse stands behind patient, about to smash an inflated paper bag). "Okay, Mr. Collins, let's see how that heart of yours is doing."

8/19/19
Well, my classroom air conditioning is now so high I almost need a sweater. #feastorfamine

Note to self: after hand sanitizing, do not immediately stick your finger in your eye, genius.

Jami: Sanit-eye-ser. You're welcome.

It occurs to me that saying that I'm 'sterilizing my students' might be open to misinterpretation. #doesn'tmeanit'snotagoodidea

I guess those are real solar tubes in my new ceiling. There's a rainbow on my whiteboard.

I now have a vampire-murdering device in my room.

8/20/19
And once again the school office has stacks of the local paper available, with a giant liquor store ad insert.

That's probably for the teachers, things being as they are.

An original First Folio of Shakespeare. (photo 95)

Who says self-publishing never works?

I'd forgotten how much work it is to talk mostly nonstop for 4 1/2 hours every day at the start of the year.

Me: Class expectations, setting up online accounts, explaining how to complete forms, fire drill procedures...

Tina: Fire Drill Procedure: If you see the instructor run, YOU run!

Me: I can only run maybe 300 steps before I gasp for air now, so I'm screwed.

Kelly: Why are you gasping for air? I thought you'd been running.

Me: It takes a really long time to get back in running shape after a heart transplant. Months or years, because of the missing nerve, etc. I'm actually starting a lot earlier than most people do.

Kristi: I was always hoarse at the beginning of the year.

Me: Getting there. Have to do it again tomorrow. Then I get 2 days of watching them do silent diagnostic writing.

Toni: Terry, I don't know how you do it. I once volunteered to teach kids about disabilities at my son's school for a two-hour slot and I was exhausted. It took almost as much energy as performing.

Me: Yeah, after the 30th year you get used to it.

Plus, this is a breeze compared to teaching violent Crips and Bloods on a moving wagon train in Klan-infested Alabama. Seriously. Check out www.VQ.com to see. #that'llbeawholeotherbooksomeday

Yeah, my classroom is fully inclusive. (photo 96)

Facebook just sent me an ad to apply to teach in MY OWN FREAKING DISTRICT!

Dave: Do they need an assistant theatre/ Shakespeare/dirty joke teacher?

Me: Don't trample on my turf, dude.

Dave: I would help further your legend and maybe get us both fired before mid-terms.

Sean: Is there something they haven't told you?

John: So...do you think you'll get the job?

Me: No, the asshole who has it refuses to retire. Something about needing health insurance, blah-blah-blah...

Julia: That's worse than Amazon emailing me to review my own book.

Me: Oh, I've had that, too.

Scott: "This author is unbelievable! It's like he's right inside my head!"

Victoria: You should apply. Just in case.

8/21/19
So much talking in class the past 2 days that I had to sit down in the last class and suck on a throat lozenge. The next 2 days are shutting up and watching them write, thank Odin.

8/22/19
Today's irony sweepstakes:
My early heart failure symptom was being out of breath climbing the school parking lot steps. Now that I'm 'cured' with the new heart, I have the same damned symptom, thanks to the missing vagus nerve, because Archie McThump-Thump isn't warmed up in the morning, after sitting in the car commuting.

Me: "I think I can, I think I can, I think I can..."

Tim: I miss my vagus nerve.

Classroom before and after. Not done yet, but usable. 60 posters & pictures hung since yesterday afternoon. #pushpinbankruptcy (photos 97, 98)

Scott: Nice, but I still don't miss it...

Garalt: You'll have a couple of newer posters from Dublin, signed by the whole company and dedicated to you.

Judging by how much my 1-hour therapeutic massage just hurt, every muscle and ligament was tighter than piano strings and knottier than a mile of tangled rope. The bike thighs, especially, hurt in Technicolor as she dug in to loosen them up. Needed to unlink everything after weeks in the hospital and months of creaky recuperating.

Me: Got out of bed feeling like I'd just played rugby...but in a good way, I guess.

8/23/19
I am happy to report that, for the first time in 30 years (howsoever brief it may be), I have NOTHING in my school e-mail Inbox.

Jim: It's an easy accomplishment if you feel no responsibility to your colleagues, parents, administration, etc. Cntl-A. Del. Done.

The Transplant Games next year will have an event — and I am NOT making this up — called 'Dancing with the Scars.'

Jim: Well, actually...I do think you are making it up.

Me: It's on their website. Read it and weep.

Julie: Do it!

Me: Oh, you don't want to see me try to dance. Transplanted hearts would fail from the horror-shock.

8/24/19
Apparently getting a full chiropractic adjustment and an aggressive therapeutic massage at the same time causes one's old body to painfully rebel at being put back where it belongs.
"And the Grinch's heart grew 3 sizes that day..." (photo 99)

Me: "Then the Who's cut it out and sliced it up."

Me: ♫"You're a dead one, Mr. Grinch..."

Facebook sent me this memory from 2017: "Had the appointment with the guy who put in the pacemaker 2 months ago today. He used the world's most expensive laptop to scope it and declare everything hunky-dory. I'm as 'cured' as I'm ever going to be. I don't have to see him for a year. Woo-hoo!"

Well, THAT was certainly a premature declaration.

8/25/19
The wife today, during a private interlude that I shall refrain from describing in any more detail, referred to my transplant scars as 'your stars and stripes.' (drainage spots and incisions)

All together now, a rousing chorus of 'The Scars and Stripes Forever.' A-one, and a-two...

Exercising my renowned social skills at the block party next door.

I survived. That's sort of a theme here.

I'm back teaching, writing, running, cycling, curling...snarking.

So...let us make this the end of the transplant memoir. If I caught a terminal infection there, what a great finish to the book it'll be. If not, I'll continue to be YOUR terminal infection, world. (photo 100)

* * * * *

That may be the end of the memoir, but not the end of the snark. I'm still rambling on these sites:

www.terrykroenungink.com (my official author site)

www.facebook.com/terry.kroenung

And please support the good work of Donor Alliance:
www.donoralliance.org

ALL JOKING ASIDE

Some sobering statistics:

The average heart transplant patient waits 144 days before finding a donor. Nearly 50% have been waiting over a year. Over 3,000 people in the U.S are on the list at any one time. A new patient goes on the list every 10 minutes. 18 die **every day** waiting for organ transplants.

I found a donor in 20 hours and went into surgery 50 hours after that. Listed on Friday, transplanted on Sunday.

Yeah. Go figure. The amount of insane luck I've had throughout this weird adventure boggles the mind. I am not unaware of it. The doctors and nurses marveled at it in front of me daily.

But not everyone has been so fortunate in this. Getting a heart transplant has one significant drawback.

Someone has to die.

This was a significant part of the pre-transplant routine, dealing with any feelings of guilt that I might have as a recipient. The team went to great lengths to assure me, as they do all other recipients, that "you're not murdering someone. They already had their misfortune and you didn't make it happen. This donor, like all others, chose beforehand to generously turn lemons into lemonade. Accept it in the spirit it is given and let them have some immortality."

I don't know who my heart once belonged to, nor his family. Someone let slip that he was from New Mexico and only 19 years old, which they weren't supposed to do. That's the extent of my knowledge. I don't even know if the donation was the idea of the young man, or if his family was forced to make a sudden decision in the face of a tragedy.

But I do know, or can at least guess, this: he, and his family, are spectacularly unselfish and incredibly brave. I waited two days after being notified that I was getting the heart, because they donated every available organ to save other people. A single donor can help 8 desperate patients. I went last because the heart was serving all those other organs until they could be removed and transported.

This year's holidays had to be awful for them: Mother's Day, Father's Day, Independence Day, Thanksgiving, Christmas, the young man's birthday. He wasn't there and that had to be a miserable gut punch. But I hope the fact that he lives on, literally, in so many other people takes some of the agony out of it. He won't be celebrating those days directly anymore, but many others, and their families and friends, will. Few people, unless they rescue people from a burning building, get to say that.

If they by chance read this book someday, I hope they understand that nothing in it is intended, in any way, to poke fun at them or my donor. This is a record of how I felt at the time, head spinning, trying to find a way to handle the situation. Sometimes I may have said something that could be interpreted as rude, or at least not in the best of taste. If anything seems offensive, I deeply apologize. I would never want to cause more pain.

It's also offered as a way for those in similar straits, particularly recipients, to identify with some of the same issues that come up in all heart transplants, and to chuckle a little at them.

Because when we laugh at life's misfortunes, we win…for a while, anyway.

Medical Terms Glossary:
(because you have no idea
what 'orthotopic allograft' means)

*I provide this glossary as a public service, since there's a lot of medical jargon in the book. Many of these were explained in the text as I went, but I wanted them all in one convenient place. The information is as accurate as I can make it. I **may** have snarked-up some of them, though. (okay, I snarked them **all** up. Happy?)*

A

Ablation: a catheter procedure to neutralize a bad electrical pathway in the heart that is causing arrythmias, generally by driving a spike into the artery next to your naughty bits and poking around literally all day.

Adhesive leads: Sticky patches stuck on your body, usually 10 of them, to measure your heart's electrical activity (ideally, you have some activity); the adhesive remains for some time after you leave the hospital, unless you own a sandblasting machine.

Allograft: a transplant of tissue/organ from someone who isn't you; not to be confused with graft, which is stealing from someone who isn't you.

AlloMap: a blood test to detect organ rejection, done in lieu of a biopsy; no, it's not a Google app.

Amyloidosis: a disease where abnormal proteins (amyloid fibrils) collect in tissue; it kills you in 10 years or less, especially if it infiltrates the heart; the most common types are AL (mutant), and ATTR (wild); my PYP test made it even more common by falsely saying I had it.

Anschutz Medical Center: Technically, the University of Colorado Anschutz Medical Campus in Aurora, Colorado, a Denver suburb; built on the old WWI Fitzsimons Army Medical Center (that place looks like a scary Soviet office building); named for the billionaire who made sure that some of his money paid for getting that name on every darned wall there; state-of-the-art medicine: this is where you go when fate has tried to utterly screw you.

Arrhythmia: abnormal cardiac rhythm, due to a wonky electrical system in the heart; makes the heart beat too quickly (tachycardia), slowly (bradycardia), or irregularly. Most aren't serious, but some are immediately or quickly fatal; I gave that last one my best shot, but proved incompetent at dying.

Asperger Syndrome: very mild autism, usually high-functioning, identified by poor social skills and extreme perseverance at particular interests/ hobbies; yes, this is why I don't look you in the eye when I'm organizing my Eeyore collection.

Athlete's heart: thickened/enlarged heart muscle and very low resting pulse, from intense and prolonged endurance exercise; makes the heart more efficient; mimics heart trouble found in a non-athletic person, so don't just assume you have it and ignore warning signs; my doctors thought this might be my trouble; they were partly right, as my heart certainly tried to set the Olympic record for weirdness.

B

Biomarker: a detectable substance that indicates the presence of a disease; cardiac markers are blood tests that ring alarm bells when they are out of the safe range and indicate heart stress; Magic Markers are indicators of parental stress from toddlers ruining your freshly-painted walls.

Biopsy: taking a tissue sample for analysis/detection of disease; in my case, poking my poor jugular vein with a wire until it chews off bits of my heart and spits them out to the lab; in another setting, it would be called felonious assault; so-named because they want to biop-see what's inside you.

Blood culture: using your blood sample to try to grow evil bacteria in the lab, to see if you have an infection; my blood is so cultured, it has season tickets to the Metropolitan Opera.

BMP: Basic Metabolic Panel, the routine blood test that looks at electrolytes, blood urea nitrogen, creatinine, and glucose; it screens for kidney problems and general overall health; Fun Fact: Russian armored personnel carriers are also called BMP's and will ruin your overall health.

BNP: Brain natriuretic peptide, a hormone in the blood which indicates cardiac stress if above the normal upper limit of 100; mine was 900, meaning my heart was beyond stressed and into the land of Righteously Pissed-Off About All of This.

Bone density scan: low-radiation test for potential osteoporosis, which the transplant medications make more likely; I'm happy to report that I am dense (hey, wait a minute…).

Borg Scale: Measure of perceived effort, during exercise, necessary for me because my denervation means I don't get the usual physiological feedback on how I'm doing; it goes from 6 (no exertion at all) to 20 (maximal exertion); used by doctors to detect how much trouble you're in as you chug away on their #$*! treadmill; also used by *Star Trek* captains to detect how much trouble they're in as they flee assimilation.

Boston Scientific: a zillion-dollar medical technology company; they made my pacemaker; they also had to pay $119 million for faulty transvaginal mesh (surprisingly, I received none of that money); naturally, their headquarters is not actually in Boston.

Bradycardia: abnormally low heartbeat, usually anything under 60 beats per minute, though each person is different; some are naturally low and not in danger, and athletes have often trained their resting pulses down via efficiency; but I'm here to tell you, blacking out and falling on your face walking your basset hound does not fit into either of these categories.

C

Cardiac episode: a polite and reassuring term for "Holy crap, my ticker's blowing up!"; covers a multitude of possibilities, most of which I got to experience on my toboggan ride toward transplant.

Cardiac stress test (V/O2): walking to nowhere on a treadmill while covered in those sticky leads and "breathing" through a tube that measures your oxygen efficiency and cardiac function; I had 2 of these that were essentially normal; 10 days after the second one, I had a heart transplant, so it's clearly more art than science; but hey, the people working in the treadmill manufacturing industry have kids to feed.

Cardiac tamponade: when fluid builds up in the pericardium, smothering the heart's pumping action; a serious, life-threatening event, especially if it happens suddenly and quickly; having endured this once, let me argue against it as a recreational choice, as the needle they revive you with (sans painkiller) is the size of Ahab's harpoon.

Cardiologists: heart doctors, those folks who wander into your hospital room with "very serious expressions", especially when nothing they've done has helped you and it's time to yank the offending sucker out.

Catheter: a thin tube inserted into your long-suffering body to pour stuff in, drain stuff out, or perform a procedure without gutting you like a fish; I'm personally responsible for the stock price rise of catheter manufacturers.

Catheter Lab: that room full of NASA-like machines where they do your biopsy, pacemaker insertion, or right-heart catheterization; usually just called Cath Lab, which sounds to me like there should be a friendly black retriever named Buddy in there.

CMV: Cytomegalovirus, basically really, really obnoxious herpes; if your immune system is on vacation, this can affect most of your organs and totally wreck you, even fatally.

D

Defibrillation: zapping your chest with enough volts to jump-start a Mack truck; they say it's to restore your heart rhythm and save your life, but I think they just love watching you flop around like a landed trout.

Denervation: lack of electrical signal transmission in a nerve; in my case, cutting the vagus nerve because that's the only way to install a new heart; now when outraged people say, "You've got some nerve!", I have plausible deniability.

Dipstick urinalysis: supposedly named this because you dip a strip of reactive pads in urine and they give results by changing color; I think it's really because you supply the sample with your own dipstick.

Diuretic: any substance that increases urination, like caffeine, alcohol, or realizing that you're about to get a heart transplant.

DSA test: donor-specific antibody test; used before transplant to better match organs with donors, and after transplant to screen for antibody rejection; not the same as body rejection, which is when she's just not that into you, dude (see 'friend-zoned').

E
Echocardiogram: usually just called an echo; a sonogram of your heart; they slather your chest with cold slime and trace a probe all over it, measuring it's function in detail; a complete one takes about 45 minutes, most of that time while they're making you hold your breath until you turn purple.

EKG: an electrocardiogram, where they put 10 of those annoying adhesive leads all over you to detect the heart's electrical signals; used to diagnose cardiac issues; pro tip: no, you can't surf a P-wave (which sounds like a plumbing problem).

Edema: abnormal fluid accumulation in your body, which usually indicates a problem; I had abnormal fluid accumulation once and had to go to a 1q2-step rehab program.

Ejection fraction: usually just called EF, this is a measure of how much blood your left ventricle is sending out to the body; it refers to the percentage of the ventricle's volume that is squeezed out with every beat; normal is around 50-65%, though there's quite a range with individuals; mine was 20% when they did my transplant; it had been 65% only a year earlier; and no, I'm not going to make an 'erection fraction' joke (they're too…hard…to come up with).

Endoscopy: specifically, esophagogastroduodenoscopy (just gave my spell-checker a stroke), sticking a flexible tube with a camera/light on the end to inspect all of your swallowy bits (esophagus, stomach, etc.); make sure your doctor uses a fresh instrument, not the one for your recent colonoscopy.

EMT: Emergency Medical Technician, those underpaid lifesavers who keep you going in the ambulance all the way to the hospital, so the Emergency Room doctor can bill you.

Etiology: this simply means 'cause', but apparently medical journals pay by the letter.

Explant: to remove from the body, like they did with my horrifying old heart, which is probably under a floor somewhere, driving someone to murder.

F

Fecal occult blood: the greatest medical test name ever; it looks for blood in your poop that isn't visible to the eye, which indicates cancer, etc.; also the greatest death-metal band name ever.

Femoral artery: the big artery that runs along your inner thigh, next to the pleasure-bits, used as a catheter entry point; one of its segments is called the subsartorial, which sounds like a slur on your clothing choices (since you're wearing an assless gown, the criticism is legitimate.

Flatline: when your heart monitor screen doesn't show those perky bouncy heartbeat spikes; this is generally interpreted as, well, 'freaking dead', to use the clinical term; the resuscitation rate isn't good for this; I've watched myself flatline repeatedly, which certainly gets lots of immediate loving attention from the nursing staff, but mine only lasted a few seconds at a time and was caused by my sick sinus syndrome (the heart's backup system would kick in each time).

Fosomax: drug used to treat osteoporosis; it wrecks your stomach; since it's alendronic acid, that should be no surprise; it's also of dubious use, since one of its side-effects is femur fractures and osteonecrosis (bone death) of the jaw; yet somehow the inventor still made big bucks off it.

G

Granulatomous: means 'containing granulomas'; are you fully informed now?

Granuloma: a grainy structure in an area of inflammation; sarcoidosis is a granulomatous condition; Granulomatous Maximus was the Roman general with the worst skin condition in the army.

H

Heparin: blood-thinner pumped through my IV to prevent blood clots and strokes; they gave me so much my blood must be transparent by now.

Hepatitis A/B: nasty inflammatory liver diseases; I was given spectacularly achy injections for them pre-transplant; I think the A stands for 'awful' and the B for 'burning.'

Holter monitor: a portable cardiac monitor worn around the neck; invented by Dr. Holter in Montana, of all places; his partner was, and I swear this is true, Dr. Glasscock (clearly he went into the wrong specialty).

Hydrogel: a Vaseliney goo used to fill and dress wounds, such as my 9 drainage tube incisions; basically spackle for the holes the Cardiothoracic Surgery Team inflicted on you.

Hypertrophic cardiomyopathy: thickened heart muscle without an obvious cause; this is what they first thought I had, until someone decided that that wasn't cool enough to write a grant proposal for.

Hypothyroidism: disease where the thyroid underproduces its hormone; I have this due to benign nodes in the gland; I take levothyroxine for it, the most commonly-prescribed medication in America (and that's where the word 'common' ceases to be applicable on my medical chart).

I

ICD: implantable cardioverter/defibrillator, a Cadillac of a pacemaker that can electrically return your heart to its correct rhythm or, if necessary, shock the hell out of it to do the same thing; they were about to put one of these in me and send me home, when the transplant rep came in and said, "Not so fast, bucko! That's not nearly cool enough for this team."

ICU: Intensive Care Unit, where they put the potentially doomed; more expensive beeping toys, more staff, more #$%@ rules for me to ignore (except for the sock color code—Odin help you if you violate that; they may violate **you**).

Immuno-compromised/suppressed: when your immune system has been locked into a chokehold by circumstance and is trying to tap out; heart transplant anti-rejection meds cause this as an intended part of treatment; the art is in balancing the two so that you don't come down with pneumonia or some other scary infection; in my case, the white blood cells were as few and far between as my high school dates.

Incentive spirometer: a rain gauge-looking thing that you suck on in the hospital to prevent pneumonia; lying around all day and/or anesthesia make you prone to lung problems, so inhaling on this like it's a lame bong helps fill your lungs all the way to the bottom; the 'incentive' is to not end up on a slab in the hospital morgue.

Infusion: fancy term for pumping you full of chemicals with an IV; related term: confusion, where you wonder why they're doing it at 2 a.m.

IV: shorthand for infusion; also the number of fingers I hold up when I want to express my displeasure with getting one, but don't want to piss off the person keeping me alive (hey, that middle finger's in there, it just has a posse).

J

Jugular vein: big vein draining blood from the head and back to the heart, as opposed to a vain juggler, who thinks **way** too highly of keeping 7 balls in the air at once while in a clown suit.

L

Left atrium: upper chamber of the heart that receives blood from the lungs and sends it down to the left ventricle; Fun Fact: atrium means 'entry hall' in Latin, though if mine had pools of blood in it, I'd have to notify the authorities.

Left ventricle: lower chamber of the heart that receives blood from the left atrium and pumps it out to the body; ventricle means 'little belly' in Latin (I wish I had one of those, but age does catch up with one); by the time of my transplant, a 'tricle' was all it put out.

Lidocaine: a drug used to numb an area before something even more awful happens to it; one side effect is irregular heartbeat, which makes me wonder why the frack they inject it into my neck before a cardiac biopsy.

LVAD: left ventricular assist device, a wearable implanted pump that keeps you alive until a new heart is found, or possibly permanently if that's how the dice fell; requires a heavy battery harness that sort of makes you look like you're packing 2 cool shoulder holsters.

M

Microbiota: the happy little microorganisms living in your digestive tract, essential for health; they prevent bad bugs from taking over, boost the immune system, metabolize drugs, and help control metabolism; some of the transplant meds, specifically antibiotics, nuke these little guys and can cause health issues; there is a **gut-brain axis**, a sort of jungle telegraph that sends signals back and forth to make things happen; it's important, despite the name sounding like the cafeteria where Nazi scientists ate; Fun Fact: there are 100 trillion microbes in there, weighing 3-5 **pounds**.

Mycophenelate: anti-rejection drug that suppresses your B cells and T cells; mine come in capsules that look like the Denver Broncos' colors (not an encouraging sign, considering their recent play).

N

Neutropenic: extremely low white blood cell count, greatly increasing the risk of dangerous infection; usually caused by suppressive meds in transplant patients; as I write this, I'm neutropenic…my white cells have been, um, neutrolyzed.

Nurse practitioner: an advanced medical practitioner, but not fully authorized to provide the services a physician does; they have advanced degrees and are very capable; those on my transplant team might as well be doctors, because I can't tell the difference—maybe it's all of that practicing ("Hey, how do I get to the Mayo Clinic?" "Practice, practice, practice…").

Nystatin: sweet yellow goo taken as a mouth rinse 4 times a day to prevent thrush infection (basically an oral yeast infection that can b e very dangerous to the immunosuppressed); I had a thrush infection in my yard, but the hawks took care of it.

O

Orphan disease: a disease so rare that it's not economically viable for private companies to spend tons of money finding cures or treatments; usually the government has to invest; guess which lucky author has one of these?

Orthotopic: a medical procedure to put something in the same place as the old one, like the typical heart transplant; Fun Fact: it was said of old Hollywood studio mogul Jack Warner: "He's a great guy. Why, he has the heart of a small boy…in a jar on his desk."

P

Pacemaker: a computer the size of a pocket watch, implanted in the upper chest, that regulates heart rhythm; you'll need it when you get the bill for the thing.

Pericardiocentesis: draining fluid from the pericardium so it won't fatally smother the heart; a much more soothing term than "Oh, my freaking god, look at the size of that needle!"

Pericardium: tough double-walled sac holding the heart; it helps prevent infection and lubricates the heart against friction as it pumps; when you have inflammation in it from a recent pericardiocentesis, acid reflux is so awful that I'd have jumped out of a window when I had it, except that we lived in a 1-story house.

Peritonitis: dangerous inflammation of the abdominal cavity; can be quickly fatal if not treated; this came with my appendicitis, but I didn't pay a lot of attention to it because all I could focus on was the doctor saying that I also had gangrene in there (prioritize when hospitalized).

Phlebotomist: the technician who cheerfully draws your blood with needles of varying size and cruelty; for my pre-transplant evaluation, mine took 20 vials of blood off of one jab—she's still my hero, considering that it could've been 20 sticks.

PICC line: peripherally inserted central catheter, for long-term infusions; I had one to pump 6 weeks of antibiotics after my pacemaker surgery; poked into my upper arm through the brachial vein, all the way to the heart; on the last day, the nurse arrived to 'take your PICC.'

Protonix: adorable diamond-shaped yellow reflux meds, so I don't end up on the floor in a fetal position begging for the sweet relief of death again; abdominal pain is potential side-effect, which doesn't even surprise med anymore.

Prednisone: everybody's #1 favorite soul-destroying steroid and immunosuppressant and the reason I have to take the Protonix; can cause psychosis, which at least gives me plausible deniability now.

PYP scan: technetium Tc 99m pyrophosphate scintigraphy (sounds like technobabble on *Star Trek:* "Captain, we've lost power to our technetium Tc 99m pyrophosphate scintigraphy! I canna maintain orbit!" "Relax, Scotty, I'll just seduce another alien maiden and all will be well."); this is a test for cardiac amyloidosis, where they pump radioactive sludge into a vein and then scan you for 30 minutes in a rotating machine that looks like it was bought at a Bond-villain auction; they had such iffy results that they had to do it to me 3 times, supposedly a first for my medical center; it was also supposedly 97% accurate…lucky me, I'm one of the 3%.

R

Right atrium: upper chamber of the heart that receives blood from the superior and inferior vena cavae (don't cry, little buddy, they told Napoleon he was inferior, too) and sends it down to the right ventricle to be pumped to the lungs.

Right-heart catheterization: similar to a biopsy, but without all that chewing and scraping; it measures pressures in the heart and pulmonary artery; if the figures are out of the norm, doctors get that Very Concerned face; I had one the first day at Anschutz; later they could check pressures through my Swan (a charming name for a scary-looking monstrosity constantly hanging out of my neck).

Right ventricle: chamber of the heart that pushes old blood out to the lungs for a breath of fresh air, and maybe a few steps for the Fitbit.

S

Sarcoidosis: auto-immune disease that infiltrates cells with granular tissue; rare in the heart, but a Very Bad Thing when it happens, as with me (80% of my heart muscle was gone); related term: Cutty Sarcoid: drinking too much of this also leads to Very Bad Things.

Shingles: yet another herpes affliction that is nasty in the immunosuppressed (can cause pneumonia); a wretched, painful rash that reappears decades after you've had chickenpox, which hardly seems fair (then again, if life was fair, my over-exercised corpus wouldn't have needed a heart transplant).

Sphygmomanometer: fancy-dancy name for a blood pressure cuff; I have literally never heard it called by its name in all of my hospital time (I think it's embarrassed because when it got in trouble as a child, its mom would holler, "Sphygmomanometer Jones! You get in here right now!").

Sternomastoid: officially called the sternocleidomastoid; the big muscle on the side of the neck that turns the head; this is what frequently aches/bruises after a biopsy, when the doctor gets too zealous with ramming the catheter in like he/she's got a hot lunch date (speaking of hot, maybe that's why the name starts with 'sterno.').

Stool: medical term for poop; makes you want to never sit on a barstool ever again.

Swan-Ganz catheter: humungous yellow neck catheter that hung out of my neck for a week after the transplant; used for measuring cardiac/pulmonary pressures, since it runs all the way down to the pulmonary artery; mine was a paired with a purple IV line not much smaller; Fun Fact: it's sometimes called 'the kiss of the yellow snake', which inspires too many dumb jokes for me to choose.

T

Tacrolimus: major immunosuppressive drug, used to decrease T cells; tiny capsules that almost blow away if you breathe on them; comes from a soil bacterium, which makes it sound a little less cool; also used, and I'm serious here, to treat dry eye syndrome in dogs and cats (just who the hell got the idea to try that in the first place?).

Thrombosis: a blood clot in a vessel; I have 2, one in each arm, from bad IV's, that still haven't resolved months later; the doctors keep telling me that they aren't a problem, they're common, they'll go away on their own, but I'm guessing if I get one in my jugular from all of the biopsies, they'll change their tune.

Tinnitus: ringing in the ears; I've had this non-stop for a decade or more; they scanned my brain for a tumor, just to be safe, and found nothing. Insert your sarcastic comment here: _____.

Transplant list: the regulated procurement system overseen by the National Organ Procurement and Transplantation Network, to keep things fair and equitable for everyone; the average wait to get a heart is 144 days, but I got mine in 20 hours, somehow; I wouldn't blame a patient who's waited a year for questioning the whole 'fair and equitable' thing, but I had nada to do with it.

Troponin: a biomarker indicating cardiac stress; this is what alerted Dr. Carlyle at my first ER visit to immediately throw me in a hospital bed and keep me there; the detectable level should be almost zero, no more than .04; mine was .25, which is apparently enough for alarm bells; immediately after the transplant, it was briefly at 57.99, which just shows you how pissed-off a heart gets when you evict it from its home with knives.

V

Vagus nerve: the longest nerve of the autonomic system; it connects to the heart for regulating pulse rate; it has to be cut to install a new heart, which is why my pulse is around 100 most if the time, and why I have to be sure to warm up before running or biking and not just dive into it; Fun Fact: women with complete spinal cord injury can still have orgasms through the vagus nerve, which just goes to show you that Mother Nature's priorities are in the right place.

Ventricular fibrillation: when the heart quivers like a leaf in a storm instead of actually beating; as this is not part of the heart's Grand Plan for Keeping You Alive, cardiac arrest, unconsciousness, and sudden death result; your survival chances even in a Cardiac ICU are only about 45%; if you aren't in a hospital when it happens, make sure you can trust your next of kin not to sell all of your stuff and run away to Cancun with your wife.

Ventricular tachycardia: too-rapid (over 120) heartbeat due to bad electrical activity in the heart; if it lasts longer than 30 seconds, it's an issue for doctors to sort out, because it could lead to ventricular fibrillation and then you're likely toast (mine lasted 2 **hours**, because that's just how I roll; the ER had to shock it back into normal rhythm); if it makes your heart stop, your chances of revival are less than 50%; commonly called 'v tach' by those of us in the cool medico-victim community.

W
Wellbutrin (Bupropion): the common anti-depressant that's my Happy Pill; one of its potential side-effects is suicide, which is a bit counter-productive if you ask me, but it's also less likely than other anti-depressants to cause erectile dysfunction, so maybe it's a wash.

ABOUT THE AUTHORS

Terry Kroenung

Despite having leapt out of perfectly functional Army aircraft, gone scuba diving with sharks, and lived with Crips & Bloods on a wagon train, and also having been paid actual money to portray both William Shakespeare and Chuck E. Cheese (though, thankfully, not at the same time), school districts have still let Terry teach their children English for almost 30 years.

Somehow a winner of the Colorado Gold Contest (*Paragon of the Eccentric*), he has appeared in 3 Rocky Mountain Fiction Writers anthologies: *Found* (Colorado Book Award winner), *False Faces,* and *Broken Links, Mended Lives* (both CBA finalists). He claims to be the only author to appear in all three, and wonders why that doesn't seem to impress anyone.

The first volume in his ongoing tongue-in-cheek fantasy series (*Brimstone and Lily, Jasper's Foul Tongue, Jasper's Magick Corset*) was a finalist in the Colorado Gold Contest and won a Bronze Medal at the Independent Publishers Book Awards. Please note that he did not get to quit his day job after such stunning success.

Visit him on the web (www.terrykroenung.com) before WordPress realizes their mistake and evicts him from their site.

Janet Smith (additional commentary & photography)

Janet has been a professional designer and costumer for over 40 years (no wonder her hands hurt) getting her Apparel Design degree from the Fashion Institute of Technology in 1972 and her BA in Theatrical Costuming in 2005. She learned to sew when she was 10 years old and will now sew only for clients willing to pay accordingly for those hard-earned degrees and years of experience (which means: retired.) She has costumed many pieces for her ever-busy husband and grandkids and when she recently moved, gave away carloads of costume pieces for free (no exaggeration.)

Living with people on the autism spectrum for most of her life, she chronicled her experience in an article in the book *Easy to Love, Hard to Live With*. Being with a person on the spectrum who needed a new heart wasn't expected, but patience is something that is always useful. That and being able to withstand puns and snarky jokes at any time of the day or night.

www.ingramcontent.com/pod-product-compliance
Lightning Source LLC
Chambersburg PA
CBHW021500090426
42739CB00007B/394